The FORGETFUL GENTLEMAN

The FORGETFUL GENTLEMAN

THIRTY WAYS TO TURN GOOD INTENTIONS INTO ACTION

NATHAN TAN

CHRONICLE BOOKS

SAN FRANCISCO

Library of Congress Cataloging-in-Publication Data:

Tan, Nathan.
  The forgetful gentleman : thirty ways to turn good intentions into action / Nathan Tan.
    p. cm.
  ISBN 978-1-4521-1352-4
  1. Men—Conduct of life. I. Title.

  BJ1601.T36 2013
  395.1'42—dc23

                          2012027506

Manufactured in China
Illustrations by Arthur Mount
Designed by Galen Smith

10 9 8 7 6 5 4 3 2 1

Chronicle Books LLC
680 Second Street
San Francisco, California 94107
www.chroniclebooks.com

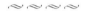

To my beautiful and talented wife, Jenny, and son, Asher, who inspire me daily to be less forgetful and more gentlemanly.

~ ~ ~ ~

Contents

≋ ≋ ≋ ≋

≋ ≋ ≋ ≋

From Bench Press to French Press: An Introduction to Gentlemanliness

MANY YEARS AGO, a "gentleman" was essentially a man of leisure. Supported by family money, investments, or property and land income, his primary purpose was attending social functions, eating well, and looking good doing it. That's no longer the case. In fact, today many of us would consider someone like that dull. This book paints a picture of a new gentleman, and provides the advice and guidance he needs to become the best version of himself as a gentleman in today's world.

Many twenty-first-century men are ready to reclaim with pride what it really means to be a man. Self-examined men who confidently know what they believe and why. Men with backbones of character and integrity. Men who aim to excel in all phases of their life—who crush it at work, prioritize family, and can always be counted on by their friends. Men who care about their health and appearance, and not simply for vanity's sake. Masculine men. Renaissance men. Men of intention, who set goals and chase hard after them. Men of knowledge, but also humility. Men who respect themselves and respect others. Modern gentlemen.

Welcome to the club.

IS THE TWENTY-FIRST CENTURY ACTUALLY THE GOLDEN AGE FOR GENTLEMEN?

Gentlemanliness is often associated with the Victorian Age, a time when men acted a certain way and were expected to act that way. Women would actually stop before a puddle and not leave a table until the men had stood up because such behavior was expected. Formal dress was required at the breakfast table. For Victorian men, acts of kindness were never acknowledged with exclamations of "Oh, what a gentleman!" or "Your mother must be proud!" To be a gentleman was to be normal. And normal is never celebrated.

Today might be the best time in history to be a gentleman. For better or for worse, gentlemanly behavior stands out today in a way it didn't in earlier times. With just a bit of effort, today's gentleman can powerfully set himself apart in business, romance, and social society, and his actions carry more significance and influence, simply because they aren't expected. You have a wonderful opportunity to invest in and impact the lives of those around you. What more could a gentleman want?

FORGETFUL GENTLEMEN AND THE IMPORTANCE OF ACTION

A Forgetful Gentleman has the best of intentions. However, when it comes to converting his good intentions into action he often struggles. Perhaps his busy, modern life gets in the way. Maybe he doesn't know how to act in a given situation or lacks knowledge on a specific topic. Or he might literally be very forgetful. Whatever the reason, it's a major issue, because we all know that being a gentleman is about action, not intention. Which brings us to the book you're holding. This is not a reference book, although it contains a lot of valuable information. It is also not an etiquette rule book, although it does address manners. This book is designed as a catalyst for gentlemanly action.

> "A truly good book teaches me better than to read it. I must soon lay it down, and commence living on its hint. What I began by reading, I must finish by acting."
>
> —HENRY DAVID THOREAU

The goal of this book is to provide you with the tools and framework to integrate its contents into the fabric of your day-to-day life. In thirty easily digestible chapters, you'll find thirty wide-ranging topics relevant to the modern man. Some of the information will be new, some of it "forgotten," but all of it is designed to help you become the best, most gentlemanly version of yourself. At the end of each chapter you'll be presented with a question to contemplate, a gentlemanly quote to remember, and an action step. Jump in! The exercises are intended to be achievable and accessible, and guide dynamic exploration of the topic at hand.

Have fun with this book, and make the experience your own. On whatever schedule feels comfortable, with friends or going solo, your approach to the information and advice in these pages is less important than the fact that it leads you to ACTION.

Now go forth and be a gentleman!

Ready, Set, Go-als:
The Gentleman's Bucket List

IN THE EARLY 1980s, shortly after selling his first business, a man narrowly escaped death by walking away from a plane crash caused by wing flap and landing gear error. As the plane went down, the man began to think about what he would do if he survived. Over the following few days, this man sat down and worked out a list of things he wanted to achieve before he died. His "bucket list" of 101 things has been his scorecard for life ever since and, to date, he has checked off 74 of the 101. As you may know, the man in question is entrepreneur, sports franchise owner, media mogul, and author, Ted Leonsis.

Ted's list is split into categories that are important to him. Here are some excerpts:

FAMILY MATTERS. #1: Fall in love and get married. #4: Take care of mother/father. #11: Have children become individuals and self-actualized, staying loving within the family.

FINANCIAL MATTERS. #12: Pay off college debts. #19: Create one billion dollars in value with an outside investment. #21: Conduct an IPO on a company I founded.

POSSESSIONS. #23: Own a beach home that stays in the family. #28: Own a great piece of art. #31: Restore an antique auto.

CHARITIES. #34: Change someone's life via a charity. #38: Give away one hundred million dollars in lifetime.

SPORTS. #40: Own a sports franchise (basketball, hockey or football). #51: Catch a foul ball. #55: Play St. Andrews. #64: Shoot baskets at Madison Square Garden or Boston Garden.

TRAVEL. #70: Go on safari to Africa. #75: Sail thru Mediterranean.

STUFF. #89: Swim with dolphins. #92: Hold elective office. #98: See the Rolling Stones.

Before we go any further, it is important to note that life is not about stacking up to Ted Leonsis or anyone else, for that matter. It's about thoughtfully considering what's most important to you and then intentionally striving after those things. A bucket list is not about content; it's all about intent. In fact, living life with intent is a defining characteristic of a modern gentleman. Ted calls it "living life on offense."

Have you ever heard someone say "I can't believe it's already ... eight o'clock ... or Friday ... or November"? It's always a bit sad to hear this phrase. What the person is actually saying is that somehow time got away from them. They didn't accomplish as much as they'd hoped and they aren't entirely sure how or why. Too often we let the inertia of life just push us along and then we're somehow surprised when we end up someplace we didn't intend.

Imagine floating down a river on an innertube. You're at the complete mercy of the water. It's easy work but the river dictates where you'll go, what you'll see, and how quickly you'll get there. Now imagine paddling a kayak on that same river. You can steer to explore new areas or avoid dangerous rocks. You can speed up or slow down. With enough determination, you might even be able to move against the flow of the river. You're in control. That's living a life of intention, and I

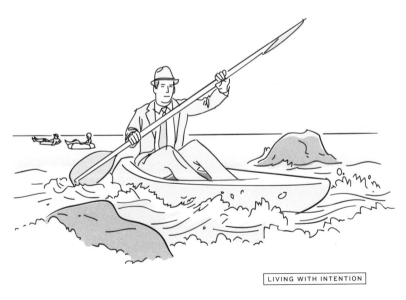

LIVING WITH INTENTION

Bucket List Tips

- Focus on immediate as well as long-range goals, social as well as personal achievements.

- Mix the audacious with the accessible.

- Have fun, and remember that the point of the list isn't to set yourself up for success with easily conquerable items but rather to provide a certain direction or trajectory for your life.

- Consider including the completion of all the action steps in this book as one of your goals.

- Once your master list is ready, create a sub-list of one-year goals—the items you commit to checking off in the next year. In some cases you might add an intermediate one-year goal that paves the way to a lifetime goal.

- Revisit your one-year list *at least* once a quarter or whenever you feel adrift, in need of direction and inspiration.

- Review both lists at the end of the year and don't be afraid to edit as your life's priorities change.

for one made the decision long ago to pick up a paddle and never say "I can't believe it's already ..." again.

One of the great things about Ted's list is how diverse and well-rounded it is. This is another hallmark of the modern gentleman. He cares about more than just himself. He is engaged with his family, his community, and the world. His interests run the gamut from sports to business to the arts. He travels. He creates. He adds value to the world. Do you?

> READY, SET, GO-ALS:
> THE GENTLEMAN'S BUCKET LIST

QUESTION TO CONTEMPLATE What does it mean to live a life of intention? What are the things in life you most want to pursue and what is keeping you from pursuing them?

GENTLEMANLY QUOTE TO REMEMBER "Don't be a spectator. Don't let life pass you by."

— LOU HOLTZ

ACTION STEP Write your own personal bucket list. Make sure your list is well-rounded by thinking in terms of life themes. You might find Ted's categories to be a good starting point.

The Proper Technique for Ironing a Dress Shirt

THE DRY CLEANER might be convenient but it's also the equivalent of hell for your fine dress shirts. Harsh chemicals, extremely high temperatures, and heavy mechanical presses can dramatically shorten the lifespan of your shirts by prematurely breaking down the fibers. And is there anything more disheartening than seeing your beautifully thick mother-of-pearl buttons return chipped and broken? The horror! It's enough to make a grown man cry.

Unless your shirt is seriously soiled, think twice before subjecting Mr. Thomas Pink or the Brothers Brooks to your local sartorial torture chamber. Launder your shirts at home and then follow these simple instructions to get the same pressed look you love and your shirts will thank you with years of service.

Hallmarks of a Fine Dress Shirt

- One hundred percent cotton is soft on the skin with none of the uncomfortable stiffness or itchiness of polyester and other man-made materials.

- Mother-of-pearl buttons replace standard plastic buttons for luxurious durability.

- The collar has roll, meaning it elegantly rolls at the fold rather than laying flat.

- The collar is substantial enough to stand tall when unbuttoned and worn with a blazer or suit jacket.

- Removable collar stays made from plastic or brass provide shape and prevent "flyaway" collar tips.

- On striped or patterned shirts, the fabric is matched such that the stripes or pattern align perfectly at seams.

- Reinforced side seam gussets (triangular pieces of fabric sewn into the bottom of the side seam) add functional durability and a bit of style should your shirt come untucked.

- Smaller, higher-cut armholes look neater and isolate arm movement to prevent the shirt body from being pulled into a disheveled mess.

STEP 1: PREPARE FOR PERFECTION

Start with a slightly damp shirt for best results. The easiest thing to do is hang your shirts after laundering them for thirty minutes or so before ironing. Set your iron to the cotton setting and let it warm up to the right temperature. If your shirt

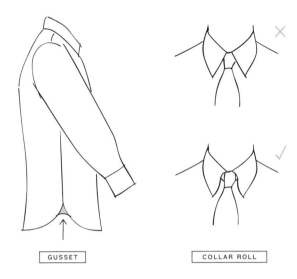

GUSSET

COLLAR ROLL

isn't 100 percent cotton, use the appropriate setting for now but seriously consider upgrading your shirt in the near future.

STEP 2: START WITH THE COLLAR

Flip the collar up and place it facedown on the board. Iron the back of the collar starting from the center and moving out to the points to avoid creasing. Turn the collar over and repeat on the outside of the collar.

STEP 3: MOVE TO THE YOKE

Drape one shoulder over the narrow end of the board and iron the shoulder piece from the yoke (where the collar meets the arm and body of the shirt) to the center of the back. Repeat on the other shoulder.

STEP 4: ADDRESS THE CUFFS AND SLEEVES

Unbutton the cuff and pull it over the narrow end of the board. Iron the cuff, removing and rotating it to each side to get to the underside. Repeat for the other cuff. Align the sleeve by pinching the shoulder seam and cuff before placing

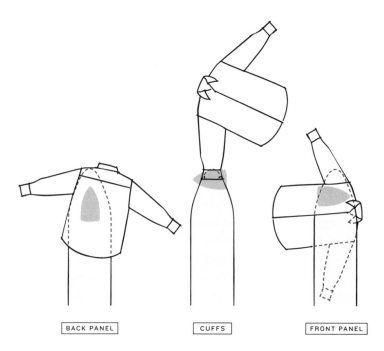

the sleeve flat on the board. Spread and smooth any overlapping fabric by hand before ironing.

STEP 5: IRON THE BACK PANEL

Drape the shirt over the board, aligning the side seam with the edge of the board. Iron as much of the back as possible, then shift the shirt so that the other side seam is aligned with the opposite board edge.

STEP 6: FINISH WITH THE FRONT PANELS

Drape one of the shirt's front panels across the board with the collar at the narrow end, aligning the side seam with the edge of the board. Iron. Pull the shirt off and then stick the narrow end of the board into the armhole for better access to the area around the top few buttons. Repeat for the other side. Always leave the largest areas for last. By leaving the front and back

IRONING TIPS

- Invest in a good iron. Rowenta makes my favorite irons and once you experience how smoothly they glide across your shirts despite their reassuring heft, I guarantee you'll be a fan as well. Rowentas warm up quickly, have accurate and responsive temperature control, and generate great steam. Upgrade to a model with an external steam tank and watch as the adjustable, pressurized steam instantly erases wrinkles.

- Depending on the hardness of your water you may want to consider filling your iron with distilled water. The minerals in tap water can build up in your iron and on your clothes. An easy test for hard water can be done by filling a plastic bottle with water about halfway (about eight to ten ounces) and adding ten drops of dishwashing liquid. Shake well. If the solution foams up immediately, your water isn't overly hard. However, if instead of foam you see a curd-like, soapy film on top of the water you probably have overly hard water.

- For stubborn creases, use steam rather than water. Steam imparts both moisture and heat at the same time and passes through the shirt instead of saturating it. This means less direct contact heat is necessary to remove the newly added moisture. Less direct heat means less wear and tear on the fabric.

- Lining your ironing board with aluminum foil beneath its fabric cover will reflect heat back into the shirt, effectively ironing it from both sides.

until last you reduce the risk of recreasing the shirt while you iron the remaining areas.

QUESTION TO CONTEMPLATE If you invest in
high-quality items, shouldn't you invest in maintaining them?

GENTLEMANLY QUOTE TO REMEMBER "You
should put on the best version of yourself when you
go out in the world because it is a show of respect to
the other people around you."

— TOM FORD

ACTION STEP Iron a dress shirt for yourself or
someone else.

Find a Mentor, Be a Mentor

TWENTY YEARS AGO, South Africa's Kruger National Park was faced with an overpopulation of elephants. The logistical impossibility of transferring full-grown elephants at that time led the park to the heartbreaking decision to euthanize the adults and save the children, who could be transported to other parks, despite concerns from rangers and veterinarians about how the young elephants would adjust. After the Pilanesberg Park game reserve received a number of the Kruger orphans, the park's rangers found that their endangered white rhinoceros population had been decimated. It turned out that the lonely orphaned elephants had grown up to be troubled teenagers.

Without the proper role models provided by a herd, the orphans had no idea of how to be an elephant and what proper elephant behavior entailed, with the young males forming a sort of "savannah gang," attacking the rhinos, and acting aggressively towards tourist vehicles. The problem was finally solved by the introduction of full-grown bull elephants into the park. The big bulls quickly reestablished the social order, and with role models in place, the younger elephants finally adapted to their new environment.

It's a harrowing story, but, there is a lesson to be learned from the elephants of Pilanesberg: guidance from those who have been there and done that can help provide the structure, discipline, and wisdom we need to thrive.

WHAT TO LOOK FOR IN A MENTOR

Seeking out a mentor isn't as easy as simply identifying the most accomplished person in your network. An ideal mentorship involves a two-way feeling-out of interest and fit. Here's what to look for when evaluating potential mentors.

EXPERIENCE. Although most mentors tend to be older, that's not necessarily always the case. Age is just a number, and in a mentor relationship, experience is what matters. Focus on finding someone with the experience you crave, not necessarily someone older than you.

CHARACTER. You should respect your mentor's character as much as his or her accomplishments and experience. Unless you share the same values, it may be difficult to see eye to eye on decision making, setting priorities, and defining success.

Where Have All the Mentors Gone?

IN YOUR NETWORK. Develop an idea of the type of person you want as a mentor and start asking around for contacts and introductions. This might be your best and most effective option.

AT WORK. Look for someone besides your immediate supervisor to be a mentor. Find someone in a position you aspire to reach one day and ask to take him or her to coffee. If available, take advantage of any formal mentor programs your employer offers.

FROM YOUR SCHOOL. Fellow alums are more likely to take your call or answer your email. You probably paid a lot for your education; it's time for some ROI.

VIA SCORE. If you're an entrepreneur, SCORE is a non-profit organization that maintains a database of tens of thousands of volunteer mentors offering help to small-business owners.

AT CHURCH. If you attend church, ask the staff for recommendations and introductions. They usually have a good pulse on the congregation and who might be a good fit for you.

FOR HIRE. You might be uncomfortable asking a complete stranger to mentor you but you might feel more comfortable offering to pay them for "consulting" work.

HONESTY. The primary role of a mentor is not cheerleader. There are many well-intentioned people without the unique skill set of your mentor to cheer you on. You seek out a mentor for advice and wisdom, the best of which is often hard to hear.

AVAILABILITY. It's great to have a business luminary as your mentor but if he or she is too busy to consistently engage with you, what's the point?

INVESTMENT. A mentor should see your potential and believe in you. Unless he or she is emotionally invested in your success, the relationship won't be as fruitful as it can be.

FOCUS. Mentors aren't just for careers. A mentor might help you be a better husband or father, golfer or spiritual leader. Regardless of the topic, make sure you set expectations so that your mentor stays focused on the area of need.

FORTUNE FAVORS THE BOLD

When Steve Jobs was in the eighth grade he decided to make a frequency counter. Lacking the proper parts, the bold twelve-year-old opened the phone book and dialed one of his heroes, Hewlett-Packard CEO Bill Hewlett. Hewlett answered the phone and, amazingly, chatted with Jobs for twenty minutes about his school project. By the end of the call, Hewlett agreed to provide the parts Jobs needed (which he personally collected and delivered) and later offered Jobs a summer job at HP, on the frequency counter assembly line!

The thing to remember about Steve Jobs, Bill Hewlett, and most other successful people is that they didn't get to where they are without help. In fact, most successful people see it as their responsibility and privilege to help the next generation of entrepreneurs, leaders, and innovators in their journey. So if you have access to someone you admire, be bold. Politely ask for thirty minutes of their time, no matter how "big time" they are, and you might be surprised at the response you receive.

A WHOLE LIBRARY OF MENTORS

Mentoring doesn't always have to be a two-way, or direct personal contact, relationship. I once asked a very successful person who his mentors were. As he rattled off recognizable name after name my incredulity rose. "Really?" I exclaimed. My friend then explained that because he grew up rural and poor, there weren't many people around who could relate to his hopes, dreams, and aspirations. Instead, he made a dream list of mentors and voraciously sought out and read every word they said or wrote. Later in life, he got to meet some of his "mentors" and thank them for the influence they unknowingly had on his life. If you don't have a mentor, head to the bookstore or check in at your local library and take your pick.

PAY IT FORWARD

No matter what stage in life you find yourself, there will always be someone struggling through a season of life that you've already been through. If you've had the good fortune of being mentored, give back by investing in another life the way your mentor invested in yours. On the other hand, if you've had trouble finding a mentor, use that as motivation to be a mentor yourself. Who knows: your mentee might open doors you never had access to before and the student might even one day become the teacher.

When looking for a protégé, look for someone who is willing, motivated, respectful, honest, and communicative. Without these elements the relationship is unlikely to be beneficial to either of you, and your efforts are best directed toward someone else. However, once you've found a protégé, invest wholeheartedly in him or her. There is great joy and satisfaction in seeing those you invest in grow and succeed.

3 FIND A MENTOR, BE A MENTOR

QUESTION TO CONTEMPLATE Is there anyone directly involved in your life that you can look at and honestly say you aspire to be like? Is there anyone in your life that can say the same about you?

GENTLEMANLY QUOTE TO REMEMBER "If I have seen further it is by standing on the shoulders of giants."

— Isaac Newton

ACTION STEP Think about what you want from a mentor relationship and, if you don't have one already, look for someone who might fit the bill. Also, consider what you might have to offer as a mentor and look into programs to give back.

A Macro View on Microbrews

MASS-MARKET BEERS are a bit like off-the-rack dress shirts, designed to generally fit everybody and therefore, by nature, not truly fit anybody. A great microbrew, on the other hand, is like your favorite indie band—too specific to ever be mainstream, but unique enough to speak to your individualized taste. Craft beer makers are shattering preconceptions about what beer can be, and thanks to a proliferation of new breweries, the experience is readily available no matter where you call home. For the gentleman beer enthusiast, this is surely a golden age.

FROM THE BASEMENT TO THE BAR

In the 1970s, the beer landscape in the United States was a monotone note of light American lager. The diverse beer brewing traditions and styles from all over the world were being pushed out by effective marketing campaigns conducted by an ever-consolidating beer industry. Indeed, by the end of the decade there were fewer than forty-five breweries left in the entire country.

Facing such dire straits, beer enthusiasts who wanted to enjoy a broader range of flavors had no choice but to brew them at home. Soon a grassroots movement of homebrews was thriving. As the quality of homebrews improved, enterprising hobbyists began sharing their creations with their local communities. Word spread, demand grew, and soon microbreweries were popping up all over the country. What started with just a handful of intrepid pioneers is now a full-fledged industry. In 1980 there were only eight microbreweries in the United States. By 1995, that number had grown to more than five hundred, and by the end of 2011 there were almost two thousand.

A similar story is unfolding in the United Kingdom where the almost forty-year-old Campaign for Real Ale has led the reemergence of real ale and traditional British beer in place of industrial lager and ale. The United Kingdom now boasts more than 550 microbreweries and the SIBA (Society of Independent Brewers) projects continued craft beer volume growth at 10 percent per year, the only segment of the U.K. beer industry on the rise. Marked by an appreciation of old-world tradition mixed with new-world innovation, it's clear that no matter what side of the pond you do your drinking on, the craft beer revolution is here to stay.

WHY CRAFT BEER?

Craft beer is an artisanal industry producing a superior product. When done with skill, you can taste the passion and care

A Microbrew Near You

With literally thousands of craft beer options available to him, the gentleman beer enthusiast is spoiled for choice. Here are twenty-four microbreweries to start you on your journey.

NORTHEAST/MID-ATLANTIC

ALLAGASH BREWING CO.
Portland, ME

BREWERY OMMEGANG,
Cooperstown, NY

BROOKLYN BREWERY,
Brooklyn, NY

DOGFISH HEAD
Rehoboth Beach, DE

VICTORY BREWING CO.
Downingtown, PA

SOUTHEAST

DEVIL'S BACKBONE BREWING CO.
Roseland, VA

SWEETWATER BREWING CO.
Atlanta, GA

MIDWEST

BOULEVARD BREWING CO.
Kansas City, MO

GOOSE ISLAND
Chicago, IL

NEW GLARUS BREWING CO.
New Glarus, WI

SOUTHWEST AND THE ROCKIES

AVERY BREWING CO.
Boulder, CO

BARRIO BREWING
Tucson, AZ

KETTLE HOUSE BREWING CO.
Missoula, MT

LEFT HAND BREWING CO.
Longmont, CO

SECOND STREET BREWERY
Santa Fe, NM

PACIFIC NORTHWEST/ CALIFORNIA

ALESMITH BREWING CO.
San Diego, CA

ANCHOR BREWING
San Francisco, CA

BOUNDARY BAY BREWERY
Bellingham, WA

DESCHUTES BREWERY
Bend, OR

FULL SAIL BREWING CO.
Hood River, OR

UNITED KINGDOM

FULLER'S GRIFFIN BREWERY
London

THE MARBLE BREWERY
Manchester

DARK STAR BREWERY, SUSSEX
Greene King, Suffolk

that goes into each batch of beer. And most microbreweries offer tours so you can actually meet and thank the malt magicians responsible for that bottle of goodness.

Some argue that good beer complements food even better than wine. While I'll leave that comparison to your discretion, there's no denying that beer pairs fantastically with many different types of food. If you're just beginning, the "heavy food/heavy beer, light food/light beer" guideline is a good starting point, but as you get more sophisticated, don't be afraid to experiment.

Need another reason to imbibe? New research is proving that there are significant health benefits to moderate alcohol consumption, including decreased risk for heart disease and diabetes. Beer is also one of the leading sources of dietary silicon, which has been linked to warding off osteoporosis.

If you live in the United States or United Kingdom, chances are, you live within ten miles of a microbrewery. Drinking craft beer is a fantastic way to support local small businesses, which are often also intimately involved in the community.

Beer culture is fun and approachable, without the pretension or snobbishness that can sometimes dampen the wine experience.

IT'S BEER O'CLOCK, HOST A TASTING

Craft beer is more akin to fine wine than it is to that tasteless, watered-down stuff you're used to drinking. The complexities and subtleties of flavor require savoring, not swigging. When you're ready for a grown-up beer experience, why not share the experience with friends?

TASTING PARTY CHECKLIST

• BEER. First, decide what kind of tasting you want to have. You might want to taste different brands of the same style of beer (e.g., a pale ale party, or a stout tasting), present a full range of different beer types (light to dark), or taste different vintages from the same brand (much like wine, some craft beer is batched, labeled, and aged by year). Once you've decided on your theme, head to your specialty beer retailer (or local brewery) and don't be shy about asking for recommendations.

• GLASSWARE. Ideally, for each guest, you want one water glass, one open-mouth taster glass for beers 7 percent ABV or lower, and one snifter-style glass for beers 8 percent ABV or higher. If you don't have access to beer glasses, wine glasses are a fine substitute. However, *do not* use pint glasses, as they won't enhance the aroma and flavor of the beer nearly as much.

• TASTING NOTE SHEETS. Make a simple placemat with room for labels and notes so that each guest can keep track of his or her drinks and thoughts throughout the night.

• WATER PITCHER. For water to drink and rinse beer glasses between tastings.

• LARGE BOWL OR VASE. For dumping unfinished beer from tasting glasses.

• PALATE CLEANSERS. Seltzer water and plain unsalted crackers work well.

• FOOD PAIRINGS. If you choose to pair your tasting with food, pick up a variety of cheeses, olives, and chocolates.

DO YOUR HOMEWORK

As the host, you should do some research on each of the beers that you're serving. Consult your local beer store and the Internet (most craft brewery websites are also a fount of knowledge). Things to know before the party: the beer's ABV (percent of alcohol by volume), brewery history, story of the beer style, and any unique or special ingredients.

DRINK AND DISCUSS

Say a few words of introduction as each beer is served. Full appreciation of a craft beer is a complete sensory experience, so ask that each guest evaluate the beer against four categories:

APPEARANCE. What do you see? Note the color, head foam, and carbonation level.

AROMA. What do you smell?

TASTE. What do you taste?

MOUTHFEEL. What does the beer feel like in your mouth?

Give everyone a chance to evaluate the beer individually and then open the group up for discussion. Above all, keep an open mind and have fun!

BEER WHISPERING

Craft brewers can be a quirky bunch, and nowhere is their eccentricity more evident than in their custom of beer whispering. If you want to join the tradition, after the initial pour but before your initial taste, hold your beer close, ask it what it wants to say, and translate the pops, crackles, and sizzles as you will.

QUESTION TO CONTEMPLATE How do you drink and think about beer in relation to wine, liquor, or even coffee? Have you been shortchanging beer?

 GENTLEMANLY QUOTE TO REMEMBER "Beer does not make itself properly by itself. It takes an element of mystery and of things that no one can understand."

— Fritz Maytag

 ACTION STEP On your next shopping trip, think twice before grabbing your usual six-pack. Spend some time perusing your grocery store or specialty beer shop and try a new microbrew. Host a craft beer tasting party to discover and explore new styles and brands with friends. The more adventurous can buy an at-home brewing kit and try their own hand as brewmaster.

Twenty Things Every Gentleman Should Own

A GENTLEMAN is not particularly interested in accumulating *stuff*. After all, money can't buy happiness, or class, and what you do is much more important than how you look doing it. However, there are certain items that, if not essential, greatly benefit a gentleman's life. The items on the following list have been selected both for function and for the activities and gentlemanly interests they suggest, and many of the items, if chosen for quality, may only need to be purchased once in a gentleman's lifetime.

A DINNER JACKET

While you may only wear it two or three times a year, the alternative to owning your own dinner jacket is plunking down two hundred dollars to wear an ill-fitting tux that some pimply seventeen-year-old sweat in all night at his prom.

With the advent of quality online custom tailors, your own made-to-measure dinner jacket needn't cost much more than a couple rentals and its addition to your closet might actually motivate you to find more excuses to dress to the nines. Tuxedos are required at "black-tie" events; either wear one or politely decline the invitation. If an event is "black tie optional, preferred, or invited," side with the host and better-dressed guests (probably about 50 percent of the men) in dinner jackets. Charity galas, opening night at the symphony or opera, and art show openings offer other opportunities to wear your tux. If you want to get even more use out of your formal wear, dress up for a nice dinner out with your significant other. Don't feel self-conscious; you'll look great and everyone will just assume you're headed somewhere fabulous. You'll probably get better service too!

A VALID PASSPORT

Nothing stirs the heart and awakens the spirit quite like traveling. Make sure you're ready for a globe-trotting adventure or a quick trip if the occasion presents itself. *Carpe diem!*

A GREAT WEEKEND SHOULDER BAG

The ubiquitous wheeled suitcase might be convenient, but it definitely lacks the romance and panache of the well-traveled, beautifully patinated leather duffel. Picture-perfect on the front seat of a convertible for an impromptu jaunt up the coast or nestled behind the pilot seat of a small prop plane descending into Cuba by cover of night, a great shoulder bag is a must-have for the jet-set gentleman. It will age with grace and is timelessly stylish, and good thing too, because if you invest in quality it'll likely outlast you.

A NAVY BLAZER

Your closet's Swiss Army knife — no other item is as versatile as the navy blazer. It complements almost any item, in any color, in any season. Opt for a single-breasted, slim, modern silhouette and, unless you're a legitimate sea captain, avoid brass buttons.

A WELL-TAILORED SUIT

Even if you work in a casual workplace, there are still many times when a suit is appropriate, if not required, dress. Slacks, shirt, and a tie might pass for "dressed up," but you're not headed to a junior high dance anymore. Isn't it time to up your game? If you only have one suit, make it solid navy or charcoal, and make sure it's been to the tailor between the store rack and your closet.

A CHEF'S KNIFE

There's no need for that unsightly block of knives taking up valuable countertop real estate in your kitchen. With some practice, a finely crafted, well-balanced chef's knife will easily accomplish 99 percent of prep tasks. A good knife will cost somewhere between a hundred and two hundred dollars, but will dice, slice, and chop faithfully for decades. Look for something between eight and ten inches in blade length from professional-grade manufacturers such as Wusthof, Global, or Shun.

A SLIM CARD WALLET

That back-pocket, George Costanza-esque wallet isn't just bad for your back; it's also killing the line of your tailored pants. You really don't need to carry every loyalty card, receipt, and membership ID you've ever received with you at all times. Get back to basics with a streamlined five-pocket card case that can be slipped into your front pants pocket or jacket breast pocket with just enough space for the essentials.

A FAMILY HEIRLOOM

Every man should have something that's worth more than its resale value. If this tradition is missing from your family, start it yourself, perhaps with an item on this list.

SOMETHING SPECIAL FOR CELEBRATING

When life's moments of joy arise, it's nice to share something to commemorate the moment. I keep a great bottle of Scotch, which is only broken out in times of celebration: after accompanying a good friend to purchase an engagement ring, following the announcement of a coworker's promotion, or with a business partner after closing a big deal.

A CLASSIC COOKBOOK

While he may not cook every night, the modern gentleman should be able to whip up a few fancy meals should the occasion present itself (e.g., a date, dinner party, or holiday). When choosing a cookbook, go with a versatile, tried-and-true classic such as *The Joy of Cooking* by Irma Rombauer, *The Fireside Cookbook* by James Beard, or *The New York Times Cookbook* by Craig Claiborne.

FINE STATIONERY

Quality paper heightens your writing experience in the same way excellent wine, delicious food, a well-built car, or fine fabric might in other areas of life. Written correspondence is an extension of your personal brand. Send a strong message by investing in distinguished letterpress or engraved, cotton-based stationery.

A WRITING INSTRUMENT

Unlike a pen, a writing instrument is not disposable, unlikely to be a corporate giveaway, and doesn't make you look like a college intern at the board table. Fountain pens are a bit fussy, but if you have the patience, the inked result can be worth the hassle. Rollerball versions offer *almost* as much class without the maintenance and impracticality.

A DEPENDABLE WATCH

Because your outfit looks incomplete without one, and because your phone is only as reliable as its battery life (i.e., not very) and checking it for the time can lead to other distractions. A "proper" watch does not run on batteries but rather an intricate mechanical movement in which the mainspring is wound manually or automatically by the natural motion of your arm. If you can swing it, get two watches, one for day-to-day/informal use and one for night/formal occasions. As a general rule, the more complicated the watch face, the less formal the watch, and leather bands are more formal than metal ones.

A DESKTOP VALET

According to my own unscientific research, over his lifetime, the average forgetful gentleman will spend over three thousand hours looking for his keys or wallet. Get precious time back and end your morning rummage routine with a desktop valet. If time is money, this may be the best investment you ever make.

A SOLID WOOD UMBRELLA

When the handle and shaft of an umbrella are made from one solid piece of hardwood, the result is strength and durability that can face a category five storm. Swaine Adeney Brigg has been making the world's best umbrellas since 1836. If they're good enough for the British royal family, they're probably good enough for you. Just don't leave this umbrella in a cab.

A PAIR OF DARK DENIM JEANS

Slim (but not skinny), straight-leg jeans in a clean, dark wash will never go out of style. Equally at home dressed up with a blazer and dress boots, or dressed down with a T-shirt and sneakers, this is how a modern gentleman does denim. The best jeans are manufactured from selvage denim, a term that refers to the clean natural edge of denim which has been woven on an old-style shuttle loom, resulting in higher quality and durability.

A PIECE OF ORIGINAL ART

One of the cues that signals the transition from "boy" to "man" and "guy" to "gentleman" is the acquisition of art. Art in this context means an original painting, sculpture, photograph, and such, not a commercial reproduction or print. Don't worry too much about things like investment potential, or provenance; just focus on what you like. Start by browsing art magazines, visiting local galleries, or going to a local art college. See shows, talk to people (artists, gallerists, students), and let your own interests be your guide. You will be surprised how easy it can be to come away with something you like, for relatively little, and even help launch a career in the process.

A PAIR OF STYLISH SUNGLASSES

If you're fishing or playing beach volleyball, a pair of mirrored sports glasses are fine, but for anything other than sports, they aren't going to cut it. While there's no substitute for trying on a few models to see what works best with your face shape, a couple styles that seem to work for most and are definitely gentleman-approved are the classic polarized Ray-Ban aviators and the tortoiseshell Persol 2720s, as favored by James Bond.

A READING CHAIR

Every gentleman needs a throne on which to relax, take a nightcap, and otherwise survey his domain. Leather is always a welcome choice, providing luxury, durability, and a strong masculine aesthetic. If you're more of a traditionalist, try a classic overstuffed wingback chair. For a more modern approach, try a mid-century style like the iconic Eames lounge chair and ottoman, part of the Museum of Modern Art's permanent collection and considered one of the most significant and collectible furniture designs of the twentieth century.

A DISTINCTIVE COPY OF YOUR FAVORITE BOOK

Get a first-edition, leather-bound, or autographed copy of your favorite book. It will make a handsome addition to your bookcase, be an interesting conversation piece, and make your reading experience even more enjoyable.

TWENTY THINGS EVERY GENTLEMAN SHOULD OWN

QUESTION TO CONTEMPLATE In your purchases, do you generally look to minimize cost, or maximize value? Can value be defined as function and utility beyond considerations of basic cost?

GENTLEMANLY QUOTE TO REMEMBER "It is the quality rather than the quantity that matters."

— Seneca

ACTION STEP Take an inventory against this list and think about adding or upgrading an item in your collection. Do your research and save up your cash. The effort and anticipation that comes before a purchase will increase the love and gratification you experience in ownership and use.

6

A Mandate to Create

AT A RECENT SOCIAL EVENT I ran into a good friend, and suddenly fell in love. Not with my friend — I'm happily married to an amazing woman — but with his beautiful, buttery soft, gray cashmere bow tie, made by the King of Cashmere, Brunello Cucinelli. I was so dumbstruck by the bow tie's beauty that its price tag — north of $400 — didn't give me any pause, until the next morning. Unwilling to let my new neckwear lust die, I resolved to find a more affordable alternative. What followed was a two-week-long goose chase that took me all over the Internet and across three different states. Exhausted and frustrated, I had a "Eureka!" moment. If I couldn't buy one, I would make one.

WORKING IN A NON-CREATION-ORIENTED WORKPLACE

Unlike previous generations, fewer and fewer modern men experience the satisfaction of tangible creation in the workplace. We move numbers around on a screen, manage people who manage other people, or sell advice, ideas, or someone else's creations. For many of us, the shift from working with our hands to working with our minds has created an unfulfilled need for connection with the physical world we live in. Physical creation (beyond the more abstract "creativity") provides that connection. A way for a man to announce to the world, simply, "I am." Creating is a primal need, but without an institutional directive to create, the internal fire to do so can flicker and die, or worse yet, we may start to believe that making things is only for certain types of people, not for us.

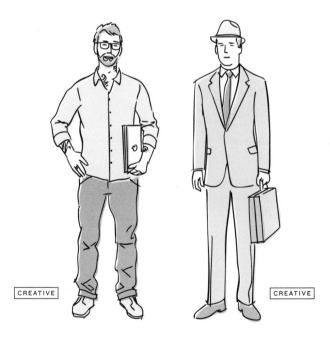

CREATIVE   CREATIVE

Everyone is creative. Everyone. You may not identify as an artist, wear thick-framed glasses, thrive amid chaos, hang out in coffee shops, or even (gasp!) use a Mac. You may not feel regularly inspired. Brainstorming sessions may make you

CREATIVITY FOR YOUR CAREER

Engaging in a creative hobby out of the office can lead to good things in the office. Here are some of the ways that a creative mindset can enhance your career:

- BETTER PROBLEM-SOLVING. Creative activities such as gourmet cooking or car restoration can help you anticipate problems earlier and envision new, unique solutions.

- MORE RESOURCEFUL. The person used to creating finds ways to overcome obstacles and dead ends. Successfully navigating the maze and minefield of the corporate world requires a resourceful and determined mind.

- RELATIONAL CONNECTIONS. Your creative hobby will give you something interesting to talk about and to potentially bond over with people who share your passion, deepening relationships and expanding your network.

- REFRESHED MIND. A creative outlet will provide fulfillment and satisfaction, relieving some of the pressure and stress from your work life. A relaxed you is a better you.

- TRANSFERABLE SKILLS. Depending on what hobby you pursue, the skills you gain might be directly beneficial in the workplace. For example, drawing ability might help you visually communicate ideas in a brainstorm session or meeting.

sweat, and you may feel straitlaced from your sensible hair-cut right down to your sensible shoes. All of this can be true, and it still doesn't mean anything. The only satisfying answer to the question "What defines a creative person?" is, simply, "Someone who creates."

The desire to create is a deeply ingrained yearning of the human soul. We all have a primal longing to bring something new into existence. The great news is that creation isn't dependent on experience, talent, resources, education, or position; anyone can create, and experience the deep sense of pride, satisfaction, and fulfillment in doing so.

EXPERIENCE, NOT ECONOMICS

Unless you're a craftsman by trade, think of your adventures in tangible creation as being more about experience than economics. Part of you may question the "opportunity cost" of making what you can otherwise buy, while your frugal side may consider DIY a way to save some money in absolute terms. While both may technically be right, both miss the point.

Think back to your childhood, before the responsibilities and pressures of life sat on your shoulders. How did you pass your time? For me, Legos were the thing. I never followed the instructions, instead dumping any new pieces into a huge tub from which I spent hours building everything from space-ships to cityscapes (but mostly spaceships). I honestly can't think of many adult accomplishments that make me feel as fulfilled as I did when I discovered how to make a plane with an operational internal bomb bay out of Legos!

When was the last time you felt the intense satisfaction of childhood creation?

GRAY CASHMERE BOW TIES, VEGETABLE INSTRUMENTS, AND MORE . . .

Once the idea that I could make my own bow tie entered my mind, I couldn't shake it. With renewed passion, I rushed over to a fabric store in Manhattan's Fashion District, armed with a pattern downloaded from the Internet and a feeling of thrilling, childlike excitement I hadn't experienced in a long time. A few nights later, I debuted my new creation at a dinner party. Most of the lines aren't sewn perfectly straight, and the hand-stitched sections in particular leave much to be desired, but I still wear my bow tie often and with pride. Wrapping the gray cashmere around my neck brings an instant smile to my face, not despite the imperfections, but because of them, and I wouldn't trade it for all the store-bought bow ties in the world.

Inspired to create something of your own but not sure what to make? Here are some projects you can start today:

- Make an article of clothing for your wardrobe. Begin by researching patterns and process in books or on the Internet to find a project you might enjoy making and having, such as a tie or bow tie (fairly easy), pair of pants (moderate), or shirt (difficult). Buy enough material to provide room for error. If it doesn't work out, try again, and appreciate the construction of your favorite clothes anew!

- Create a handmade piece of furniture. And no, assembling a flat-pack Ikea bookcase doesn't count. Bonus points if you source and utilize reclaimed wood.

- Draw, paint, or sculpt something. Hang it up or throw it away. Do it again.

- If you have a yard, start a landscaping project. Think about the areas that have promise or need help, and about how you will enjoy the results of your labor when you've finished.

- Try brewing your own craft beer, wine, or liquor. If the result is worth sharing, design your own label and gift it to friends and family.

- Prepare a home-cooked meal from ingredients that you have sourced yourself. Whether by hunting, fishing, oyster digging, lobstering, foraging, or gardening, there's nothing more delicious than a meal made from food you've gathered yourself.

- Protect your cash and portable electronics with a handsome, handmade wallet, phone, or tablet case.

- Make music with a DIY instrument, such as a cigar box ukulele or vegetable ocarina. Your carrot clarinet skills might lead to a gig with the Vegetable Orchestra, a Vienna-based ensemble that performs worldwide exclusively using handmade vegetable instruments.

- Lights, camera, action! Make a short film. These days all you need is a cell phone and a computer. Consider entering an amateur film competition hosted by your local city or filmmaking club. Even if you don't make a dime, as long as you don't spend millions on production, your film will be more successful than the majority of Hollywood flicks!

- Revisit your favorite childhood creations. Don't be surprised if Legos, Tinkertoys, and model train sets still offer the same fun and fulfillment.

QUESTION TO CONTEMPLATE Is there value in creating things yourself? How do you view things that you have made versus things you have bought? Do you ever feel dissatisfied, unfulfilled, or unsure of the impact of your work or life? How do you normally address those feelings?

GENTLEMANLY QUOTE TO REMEMBER "It is better to create than to be learned, creating is the true essence of life."

— BARTHOLD GEORG NIEBUHR

ACTION STEP Create something! If you aren't immediately inspired try this exercise: Make a list of the things that you either need or want, around the house, in your closet, or for someone else. Review your list and see if there is anything you can check off using your own two hands and a bit of ingenuity.

The MAN-icure: Masculine Hygiene

WHEN THIS BOOK was still just a concept, I asked everyone I knew, "What are the topics every modern man needs to read about?" While I spoke to both men and women, an overwhelming number of the fairer sex listed hygiene among their chief concerns. It's telling that not one man I spoke with suggested hygiene as a potential topic.

As men, many of us have this outdated notion that anything more than bar soap and a splash of water on the face is unmanly. My wife thinks that we keep telling ourselves this self-perpetuating lie to vindicate our own laziness. If I'm honest, there's probably some validity to that in my own life, but I think it goes deeper. Regardless, it's time for men to face the truth, which is that in our modern era, even if your work is labor-intensive, the male archetype no longer has rough, sandpaper hands and an etched, weathered face (especially if you don't have the age or life experience to match). And the truth is that it's near impossible to claim the mantle of gentlemanliness without caring for personal hygiene.

EYEBROWS: "IT TAKES TWO TO MAKE A THING GO RIGHT . . ."

In Victorian times, Italian criminologist Cesare Lombroso popularized a theory of anthropological criminality that stated that criminality was inherited, that criminals were born and not made, and could even be identified by certain physical traits. One of the defining physical traits of a "born criminal" was the unibrow.

Over a century later, the unibrow is still a serious crime, but the modern man has an easy get-out-of-jail-free card. Plucking or waxing the rogue hairs is easily accomplished, at home or by a professional aesthetician. Shaving between your eyebrows, however, is ill-advised, as the hair will grow back thicker, darker, and faster, requiring daily maintenance.

Pluck your stray eyebrows after a shower when your pores have opened, and pull in the direction the hair grows. Your eyebrows should end roughly in a straight line up from the inside corner of each eye, so pluck everything between. Make sure you grab one hair at a time and don't go overboard; the intent is to tame, not shape, your eyebrows. Alternatively you could have a professional aesthetician (ask at a salon or spa) wax around your eyebrows for a cleaner, longer-lasting result (good for about six weeks). Either way, once you've got a nice separation, run a beard trimmer with guard attached across the full brow to trim everything down to an even level.

NAILED IT!

Being a man means getting your hands dirty from time to

time. Tinkering with car engines, table saws, and planting beds is sure to result in some dirt under your nails. But when it's time to trade the tool belt for your work briefcase, dirty, untrimmed nails show a lack of care. If you aren't convinced people notice dirty nails, think about how many times you talk with your hands, shake hands, or pass things by hand throughout your day.

Trim your fingernails weekly and scrub beneath your nails regularly with soap and a nailbrush. Follow up with a post-shower hand lotion to keep your skin and cuticles smooth and hydrated. Better yet, treat yourself to a professional manicure. Male-only salons and spas are popping up all over, which means you can have your nails attended to while sipping scotch and catching up on sports highlights or the latest market news, all in the comfort of a leather-and-wood enclave of manliness.

Toenails often fall victim to "out of sight, out of mind" syndrome. However, the same routine should be observed in terms of nail trimming and brushing. And while you might be apprehensive about a professional pedicure, I can assure you that thirty minutes of glorious foot massaging after a long day's work will quickly change your mind.

DIRTY MOUTH?

You watch the calories you put into it and are careful about the words that come out of it; give your mouth itself the same attention and care. Brush at least twice daily, more frequently if you smoke or drink a lot of coffee, tea, or red wine. Floss daily before your nighttime brush and follow each brushing with a vigorous rinse of mouthwash. Keep an extra toothbrush, tube of toothpaste, and mouthwash at the office to freshen up before an important meeting or after a garlic- or onion-laden lunch.

Most men brush much too aggressively, which can lead to enamel wear and gum recession. Always opt for a soft-bristle toothbrush and try holding your toothbrush solely between your thumb and forefinger—you don't need any more pressure to clean effectively. Finally, don't forget to brush your tongue and the inside of your cheeks, where smelly bacteria can also accumulate.

Throughout the day, gentlemen keep their breath fresh with strong mints or breath freshener strips, leaving the bovine-esque chomping of gum for teenagers and the less well-mannered.

SKIN IN THE GAME

Human skin is an amazing thing. We have our skin to thank for protection, water and nutrient storage, temperature regulation, and the sensation of touch. Every five square centimeters of human skin can contain up to six hundred sweat glands, twenty blood vessels, sixty thousand melanocytes, and over a thousand nerve endings. Thank your skin for everything it does for you by cleansing and moisturizing it daily, and your skin will reward you with many more years of glowing health and luster.

Wash your face in the morning and again at night with warm water. Hot water can dry out your skin. Use a specific face cleanser, not the same stuff you use on your body, which is too harsh for sensitive facial skin. Select a cleanser suited to your skin type: normal, oily, or dry, and use a separate gentle exfoliating scrub once a week to remove dead cells from your skin. When you cleanse or exfoliate, you strip the natural oils from your skin, so make sure to moisturize immediately. Like facial cleansers, face lotions are different than body lotions and developed specifically for your mug. Look for something light and fragrance-free with included SPF protection.

When skin ages, the collagen and elastin fibers that are responsible for holding the skin in place break down. When skin is dry, the loosening process is accelerated, resulting in premature wrinkles. In addition to moisturizing, proper hydration of your skin can keep the inevitable at bay for years. Drink plenty of water. No need to down the fabled eight full glasses a day, but do drink whenever you are thirsty — your body's thirst mechanism is well-tuned and will let you know when you need hydration.

NOSE-Y PARKER

Due to unexplained hormone changes, as men approach and pass thirty they often find a surprising new midlife partner: dark, thick, protruding nose hair. Creeping nasal growth must be pruned back swiftly and mercilessly with a pair of round- tipped scissors or an electric nose hair trimmer. Do not tweeze nose hairs; it's painful and can lead to lesions susceptible to infection.

If you have a cold or allergies, carry a pack of tissues with you and stock your office and home with larger boxes. Blow your nose regularly, and when with company, discreetly excuse yourself before clearing your passages. No one will begrudge your brief absence from a meeting or meal if it means relief from your incessant sniffling. Never put used tissues anywhere but in the garbage or your pocket. Even when you are perfectly well, carrying a small pack of tissues can provide you with opportune "knight in shining armor" moments to help the less prepared deal with an errant sneeze.

Speaking of noses, always use deodorant, and if you use cologne, don't overdo it—one spray into the air at neck height, which you walk through rather than spray directly on yourself, should be enough. Despite clever marketing, body spray is not cologne, and makes you smell like an adolescent. Buy a real scent (hint: it comes in a bottle, not a can) and make sure to try it first as the effect can change depending on your skin and pheromones.

I'M ALL EARS

Don't make the mistake of thinking that just because you can't see into your ears, no one else can either. Clean inside your ears with a quick cotton swab swipe after you get out of the shower and, if necessary, carefully trim any unsightly protruding ear hair with a pair of rounded point scissors and the help of a good mirror.

7 THE MAN-ICURE: MASCULINE
HYGIENE

QUESTION TO CONTEMPLATE Where does hygiene rank on your life's priority list? Why does hygiene matter?

GENTLEMANLY QUOTE TO REMEMBER "Cleanliness becomes more important when godliness is unlikely."

— P. J. O'Rourke

ACTION STEP Personal hygiene can be a hard subject to broach with others. As the potential offender, it can be difficult to notice our own hygiene indiscretions, and the people we affect are often too uncomfortable to bring up the subject on their own. Do everyone a favor and take the initiative to ask a trusted friend for his or her honest opinion on your hygiene (breath, body odor, appearance). It can be a humbling conversation, but you'll get the feedback you need and give your friend the relief of saying something without having to be the one to bring it up.

iGent: Etiquette for the Digital Age

As THE CLOSING MOMENTS of Mahler's Symphony no. 9 approached, the New York Philharmonic audience leaned forward in their seats, straining for the sublime, soft, delicate notes. And then it happened. The jarring, unmistakable iPhone Marimba ringtone reverberated through the concert hall. As the ringtone played on and on, conductor Alan Gilbert did the almost unthinkable. He stopped the performance.

How does one person hold one of the world's finest concert orchestras, one of its most acclaimed conductors, and hundreds of people hostage? Technology. Or more accurately, a mismanagement of technology. In many ways, the digital age has brought with it innumerable new etiquette challenges, and at such a rate that etiquette rules and guidelines have struggled to keep pace. The result is a world of new, commonly accepted social norms developed without much careful thought, and new social situations many of us aren't equipped to deal with. What is the tech-embracing gentleman to do?

PRIORITIZE SOCIAL LIFE, NOT MEDIA

I once had a boss who would routinely call me into her office, start talking, and then leave me sitting in awkward silence while she took the phone calls and replied to the emails that interrupted our conversation, often mid-sentence. Inevitably, a topic we could have discussed in five uninterrupted minutes routinely took up to thirty minutes of piecemeal communication to get through. Although I choose to think it was not my boss's intention, I'll never forget how those meetings made me feel so unimportant and disrespected.

As a general rule, prioritize your social interactions by their proximity to an immediate, physical connection. The person you are with face-to-face has priority over the person who is calling you. Likewise, a person on the phone takes precedence over the person who is emailing, texting, tagging, or poking at you. This hierarchy allows you to be fully present in your relationships, giving them the attention they deserve. The next time you're out to coffee with a friend, put your phone on vibrate mode and let your voicemail system do its job.

As with any guideline, there are exceptions to the rule. For example, if your wife could go into labor at any moment, you'll be excused for interrupting a conversation to answer the phone. If you're expecting an exceptionally important call or email in social company, the polite thing to do is preface any conversation with a heads-up to the group and ask permission to check your phone occasionally for updates. When checking your phone, do so quickly, discretely, and never while speaking or being addressed directly in conversation.

THE NEED ... THE NEED TO PROOFREAD

According to research published in the *Journal of Personality and Social Psychology,* we misunderstand the tone of email 50 percent of the time. This is understandable, as email is communication absent of facial expressions, tone of voice, and body language. However, this is not an excuse for sending unclear or potentially offensive email. Take the time to reread your message before hitting send to ensure your words are communicating exactly what you want to say.

Proofreading is especially important on a mobile device where small keyboards, sensitive touchscreens, and diabolical auto-correct features can conspire against you. Some people have taken to adding an auto-signature to messages sent from mobile devices such as, "Sent from my mobile device, please excuse brevity, spelling, grammar." However, I think that's a bit like saying, "Sent from my mobile device, either you're not important enough to me or I'm too lazy to proofread this message."

As a gentleman, be acutely aware that all communication is a direct reflection on *you.* Don't let typos, malapropisms, or grammatical mistakes send the wrong impression.

AN iGENT DOESN'T SHOUT OR "LOL"

Typing in all caps infers shouting. A gentleman doesn't shout at people in spoken conversation and shouldn't in virtual conversation either. If you want to add emphasis, underline, bold, or italicize the word(s) instead. And please end the madness with Internet acronyms. There's nothing gentlemanly about "rotflmao," in real life or text messages. You're not a teenage girl, so stop typing like one.

THE INTERNET IS A PUBLIC SPACE

Unless you intentionally hide it, content on your social networks is fair game for HR departments. In fact, there are now numerous stories of people who have been fired for the content of their online profiles. HR reps aren't the only people looking at your profile critically. So are your friends and family, coworkers and bosses, clients, and customers. Here are some ways to ensure your social media presence works for you, not against you:

- Don't get too personal or overshare. Status updates and comments are meant for short, general statements and well wishes. Anything more personal needs to be taken out of public view to email or, better yet, offline communication.

- Some social networks allow you to group your "friends" while others provide targeted privacy settings. Take advantage of these features to separate your nine-to-five from your five-to-nine.

- Always ask permission to post and tag pictures of other people. Never post a picture the people depicted wouldn't post.

- Every detail of your life isn't worthy of sharing with the world. Don't overload other people with pointless minutiae.

- Know the difference between friends and "friends." Don't "friend" someone you don't know or hardly know.

- Be careful with apps that share information about what articles you read or which sites you visit. Your decision to read up on the latest celebrity gossip is questionable enough already without broadcasting your embarrassing reading habits to the rest of the world.

- Don't spam your friends with app invites. No one really wants to join your mafia crew or move onto your animal farm.

- New web services such as BrandYourself.com allow you to control your online reputation via search engine optimization, pushing up favorable results and helping people find you, not the drug dealer who happens to share your name.

BEHIND EVERY SCREEN NAME IS A REAL PERSON

People can become emboldened by the anonymity of the Internet to say and do things online that they would never dare do in the real world. Don't say anything via email or online post

---

Netiquette Glossary

TROLL: Someone who surfs the Internet looking to stir up trouble by posting antagonizing or incendiary comments or messages, often hidden behind an anonymous screen name.

FLAMING: Rude emails, comments, or posts intended to provoke confrontation and argument.

SPAM: Any message or solicitation sent to large groups of people without consent via email, online messages, SMS, or social networks.

CYBER BULLYING: Using the Internet to harass, intimidate, embarrass, or put down others.

---

that you wouldn't feel comfortable saying to someone face to face. If you disagree with someone or something online, handle the situation with the same grace and dignity you would offline, no matter how strongly you feel about the topic, or how poorly the other person may be behaving or may treat you in return. Remind yourself that you're dealing with a real human being, even if all you see is a screen name or avatar.

WATCH YOUR "PHONE VOICE"

Early models of the telephone required the user to literally shout into the microphone in order to be heard clearly. While technology has obviously advanced by leaps and bounds, it seems many humans haven't kept up. We've all been trapped in a public place while our ears are assaulted with lurid details about illicit love triangles, insipid conversations about what to have for dinner, or even presumably sensitive corporate information. The bottom line: have the self-awareness to realize where you are and how loud you are speaking. Don't talk on the phone in public places like airports, coffee shops, or restaurants; step outside or excuse yourself to the lobby where you won't disturb anyone. Likewise, keep phone conversations on public transport as quick and quiet as possible.

MEDIA MANAGEMENT

Mobile computing means we can now take our media on the go, 24/7. However, be careful about watching adult content in public places, especially if children are around. If you're sharing an airplane row with an eight-year-old, it may be best to watch your mature HBO drama once you get home. Also, be careful about the volume of the media coming through your headphones. The last thing anyone wants to hear on their long commute home is the thumping bass of your club music.

QUESTION TO CONTEMPLATE Do you act in the same way online as you do offline? Does your online profile deliver the same first impression as an in-person introduction? Does technology make you more or less gentlemanly?

GENTLEMANLY QUOTE TO REMEMBER "It has become appallingly obvious that our technology has exceeded our humanity."

—Albert Einstein

ACTION STEP Conduct an audit of your online presence. Look at your social network profiles as a prospective employer, father-in-law, or parent. Check every photo that you are tagged in. Read old emails and text messages for politeness, clarity, and content. Take any necessary steps to ensure your virtual persona matches your real-life character and values.

The Proper Care and Feeding of Dress Shoes

As GENTLEMEN, we clearly understand that how we dress sends strong signals to the rest of the world about who we are and what we believe. We also know that our shoes do a lot of that talking for us. As a visual endpoint, shoes attract a disproportionate amount of attention in the visual snapshot others use to create a first impression. Perhaps no other element of a man's wardrobe is more scrutinized or more important. High-quality, well-maintained shoes communicate an appreciation for value, attention to detail, and personal style, all hallmarks of the modern gentleman.

However, owning a good pair of dress shoes is only the first step in a lifelong commitment to putting your best foot forward. Getting the most out of your investment will require continued maintenance and care.

LEATHER'S ARCH NEMESIS

When it comes to leather shoes, moisture is kryptonite. And when it comes to producing moisture, feet are the body's pound-for-pound champ. With over 250,000 sweat glands, more per square inch than any other body part, your feet are capable of producing half a pint (or one cup) of sweat a day. All that moisture softens a shoe's leather sole, causing it to wear much more quickly than normal. Too much moisture also breaks down the leather upper and lining. Without proper care your shoe will literally rot from the inside out. In the face of such potent podal perspiration power, it might seem like your fine shoes are destined to die a slow, wet death. However, take heart — there are a few strategies and even a secret weapon or two that can aid your valiant cause.

THE SHOE DEFENDER'S ARSENAL

Shoe trees are shoe-saving devices made from aromatic cedar wood, formed to the size and shape of a foot. When placed inside of a shoe, this vital tool absorbs moisture and provides the necessary structure for a shoe to regain its original shape after a long day of abuse. Cedar naturally deodorizes as well, maintaining the rich new leather smell we love, and saving loved ones from our infamous "swamp foot." Shoe trees are inexpensive purchases that will pay for themselves over and over again.

Using a shoehorn when putting on shoes will keep your heel from crushing the counter (the vertical part of the shoe that wraps around the back of the foot). Although shoehorns are available in precious metals, animal horn, and other exquisite materials for the millionaire shoe aficionado, functionally there's no need to spend a lot on a shoehorn. Good shoe manufacturers and retailers often offer complimentary plastic shoehorns that work just fine. Otherwise you can pick one up for a few bucks.

What Are "Proper" Dress Shoes?

Good dress shoes are constructed completely from high-quality leather, including the upper, lining, and sole. Why? Leather breathes. Rubber soles and synthetic leathers do not.

The leather sole should be stitched, or welted, to the upper. This allows the sole to be easily removed and replaced once it has worn out, extending the life of the shoe almost indefinitely.

Even with a well-trained eye, it can be difficult to judge the quality and durability of an unknown shoe when in pristine, new condition. Rely on two criteria: price and make. For a good-quality, welted calfskin shoe, expect to pay at least three hundred dollars at full retail. If that price tag is out of reach, wait for sales or visit an outlet rather than pay full price for an inferior product. As a starting point, Alden, Allen-Edmonds, Cheaney, Church's, Crockett & Jones, Edward Green, Grensen, and John Lobb are all trusted and reliable makers of high-quality, long-lasting welted shoes.

To ensure a comfortable fit, shop for shoes late in the day after your feet have had a chance to swell naturally. Wear dress socks and make sure you try on both shoes, as your feet are probably slightly different in size. If a shoe is not comfortable in the store, it's unlikely to "break in," no matter what the sales associate might suggest.

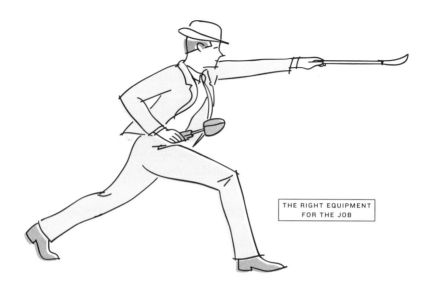

THE RIGHT EQUIPMENT
FOR THE JOB

YOUR SHOE RACK IS A BULLPEN

Just as baseball pitchers need to be rotated to perform at peak efficiency, shoes need rest between outings. Shoes should never be worn on consecutive days but rather stored with shoe trees and allowed at least forty-eight hours of respite following each use. Two pairs of dress shoes, to be alternated daily, are an absolute minimum. A well-cared-for shoe rotation of five to seven pairs will easily see its owner through a decade or two. By contrast, one pair worn daily would be lucky to see its first birthday, regardless of initial quality.

CLEANING IS CARING

Keeping dress shoes looking sharp is an easy task and a ritual you might start to enjoy once you catch the shoe bug. While paying for a professional shoeshine is certainly a valid option, for many there is a unique satisfaction in caring for one's own shoes with one's own hands.

THE DIY SHOESHINE

CLEAN: Use a horsehair brush, followed by a moist cloth, over the surface of the shoe to remove any dirt or grit. The little pieces of mineral grit that unavoidably collect on your shoes can be quite sharp and you want to avoid polishing them into the leather.

CONDITION: Use a cloth to apply a leather conditioner/cleaner. Let the conditioner dry for three to five minutes before moving on. I recommend Saphir Renovateur, a French product capable of leather miracles with a well-documented reputation among shoe aficionados as providing the world's best all-purpose shoe care.

POLISH: Apply a medium-thick coat of correctly colored wax polish to the upper using a cloth or small horsehair polish brush. When in doubt, err on the side of more polish. Remove excess wax using a larger horsehair shine brush. While Saphir makes a fantastic range of polishes, the more common and familiar Kiwi products are great as well.

SHINE: Apply a touch of water to a clean cloth and buff the wax finish to a nice gloss. A common mistake is using too much water. Fill a container with just a few millimeters of water and then dab your cloth in quickly.

THE MIRROR SHINE (OPTIONAL): Achieving the Holy Grail of shoe care requires patience and discipline, but if you can accomplish a mirror shine it will truly set you apart (unless you're in the military, in which case it probably loses some of its luster). The trick to achieving a mirror shine is very thin layers . . . and lots of them. A common misperception is that you are actually shining the leather. In reality it is the substantial coat of wax, applied in thin layers, that can be buffed to shiny perfection.

Take a polishing cloth, wrap it tightly around a finger, and add a single drop of water followed by a tiny dab of polish. Apply the mixture to the toe of the shoe using small, circular swirling motions. Repeat. You might need fifty-plus layers to achieve the full effect. As you get to the end of each layer, breathe warmly on the leather before the last few swirls. When you can tell time from a watch in the shoe's reflection, you're done.

Note: A mirror shine is only recommended for the toe of the shoe. Applying a mirror shine to flexible leather can lead to unsightly cracking.

THE PROPER CARE AND FEEDING OF DRESS SHOES

QUESTION TO CONTEMPLATE In their current state, what story do your shoes tell others about you? What do you want your shoes to say about you?

GENTLEMANLY QUOTE TO REMEMBER "A man hasn't got a corner on virtue just because his shoes are shined."

— ANNE PETRY

ACTION STEP Shine your shoes, either professionally or at home using the step-by-step instructions from this chapter. We'll work on your virtues later.

Books Every Gentleman Should Read

A GENTLEMAN doesn't gain knowledge for knowledge's sake, but rather to influence and improve the world around him. Unless leading to action, knowledge has little worth. In *Some Thoughts Concerning Reading and Study For a Gentleman,* philisopher John Locke identifies the importance of reading to the gentleman, not merely for entertainment, but for understanding. In today's digital, media-saturated world we consume a lot of "content." But the reading Locke advocates is a deeper and more introspective experience than flash downloading the day's headlines in 140-character blurbs.

If he were here today, I'm sure that the twenty-first century Locke would challenge us to slow down and bring more deliberation to our reading, both in content and in practice.

What follows is a highly subjective, decidedly incomplete list of recommended reads for the modern gentleman. As a starting point, this list will help you think about the intricacies, challenges, and triumphs of being a man that will hopefully lead to better understanding, knowledge, and, most importantly, action.

THE COUNT OF MONTE CRISTO
ALEXANDRE DUMAS

Dumas shows us the best and worst sides of a brilliant, cunning man in this ultimate tale of betrayal and revenge. Filled with adventure, suspense, and drama, this is eventful fiction at its very best. Even at 1,400-plus pages, once you pick it up, good luck putting it down.

THE ODYSSEY
HOMER

The epic journey is a theme close to the essence of manhood, and there is no journey more epic or wrought with trials, revenge, destitution, and perseverance than Odysseus's gallivant across the ancient Mediterranean.

"Reading is for the improvement of the understanding. The improvement of the understanding is for two ends; first, for our own increase of knowledge; secondly, to enable us to deliver and make out that knowledge to others. The latter of these, if it be not the chief end of study in a gentleman; yet it is at least equal to the other, since the greatest part of his business and usefulness in the world is by the influence of what he says, or writes to others."

—JOHN LOCKE

DAVID MCCULLOUGH

This book is historical literature captivatingly brought to life. McCullough provides illuminating perspective into an oft-overshadowed political figure who was every bit the equal of Thomas Jefferson, Benjamin Franklin, and George Washington. In fact, a gentleman can learn a lot from Mr. Adams, whose conduct was in stark contrast to that of his pal, Mr. Jefferson (slave owner, womanizer, hedonist, and, ultimately, mega-debtor). McCullough tells a story of intelligence, passion, romance, adventure, and patriotism, and more than anything the story of a real man. John Adams — a gentleman of the first order.

ZEN AND THE ART OF MOTORCYCLE MAINTENANCE
ROBERT PIRSIG

How can one distinguish "good" from "bad"? What is the definition of "quality"? Never have such complicated philosophical questions been so interestingly and relevantly presented. This story of the author's cross-country motorcycle trip and his thoughts from the open road is ideal for the gentleman searching for balance between "living in the moment" and pragmatic rationality.

HOW TO WIN FRIENDS AND INFLUENCE PEOPLE
DALE CARNEGIE

The advice and examples from this 1934 publication are as applicable today as they were over seventy years ago. A practical, masculine "self-help" book if there ever was one, *How to Win Friends and Influence People* will help you get ahead

LEARN TO READ THREE BOOKS A DAY

Teddy Roosevelt was a voracious reader. While in the White House he regularly read a book before breakfast and often two more after dinner. Historians estimate his lifetime reading roll in the tens of thousands. Teddy's secret? He mastered the speed-read.

Much of the joy in reading is found in carefully soaking up the purposefully articulated language of the author. There are certain times, however, when quickly downloading information is the priority. If you want to match Teddy, page for page, you'll need to learn the techniques of speed reading.

• Stop reading aloud, in your head. By mentally pronouncing each word you limit your reading speed to how quickly you can move your mouth.

• Up to 30 percent of reading time is wasted rereading content. Using your finger or a pen to underline the words as you read can keep your eyes on track and moving forward.

• Train your peripheral vision to read more than one word at a time. Practice reading lines in a book beginning three words in and ending three words in from the last word.

in business, deepen your relationships, and unleash the full potential of your life.

THE ALCHEMIST
Paulo Coelho

The modern gentleman lives with purpose and intention. *The Alchemist* is a tale about a quest for worldly treasure that becomes a journey of self-discovery, and the importance of finding and fulfilling one's own "Personal Legend." Inspirational and empowering, this book will challenge you to trust your heart, open your eyes to the universe's hidden clues concerning your purpose, and chase your dreams. After all, as the young protagonist Santiago learns, "To realize one's destiny is a person's only obligation."

INTO THIN AIR
John Krakauer

Climbing is a rite of boyhood. But while most of us left the jungle gym for the corporate ladder long ago, others graduated from hills to mountains. Krakauer offers a powerful account of his time at "the roof of the world" during the fateful 1996 Everest disaster that ultimately claimed the lives of eight climbers. The adventure will have you on the edge of your seat, even if your feet never leave the ground.

DRESSING THE MAN
Alan Flusser

The definitive guide to timeless gentlemanly style (not to be confused with fashion, which changes from season to season), *Dressing the Man* is a veritable encyclopedia of sartorial knowledge. The book's lessons are beautifully brought to life by photographs of the likes of Cary Grant, Humphrey Bogart, and the Duke of Windsor, along with side-by-side comparisons of how various color palettes work with different complexions and body types. A must-read for any gentleman who wears clothes.

FOR WHOM THE BELL TOLLS

ERNEST HEMINGWAY

Set during the Spanish Civil War, this is considered one of the greatest war novels ever written—a captivating investigation into the core of who a man is and what he holds most dear, as brought to light in the face of his mortality. This book is for any man who has wondered at what would be revealed by the crucible of war and the difference between living well and dying well.

CATCH-22

JOSEPH HELLER

Few literary quotations or titles have penetrated the common vernacular like the phrase "Catch-22," and few books have managed to dance the tightrope of satire, philosophical excursion, and comedy quite like Joseph Heller's masterpiece. If you like to think and laugh at the same time, you are a man who will love *Catch-22.*

RICH DAD POOR DAD

ROBERT KIYOSAKI

My first copy of *Rich Dad Poor Dad* came from my own dad, sent to me while I was a pre-med college student. A week later I switched majors from Biology to Business and two months following that I started my first company. Compelling, empowering, and approachable, Robert Kiyosaki's perspective on financial literacy will teach you the difference between working for money and putting money to work for you. If you, like me, prefer the question "*How* can I afford this?" to "*Can* I afford this?" then you can't afford not to read this book.

BOOKS EVERY GENTLEMAN SHOULD READ

QUESTION TO CONTEMPLATE Think about the content you read on any given day and break it down into categories: mindless entertainment, work, functional information, personal correspondence, and advertising. How much of the content you read requires deliberate thought and influences how you live life?

GENTLEMANLY QUOTE TO REMEMBER "The man who does not read good books has no advantage over the man who can't read."

— Mark Twain

ACTION STEP Choose one of the recommended titles or another book of your choice and commit to reading it with a fellow gentleman. Meet to discuss how the book impacted you and its implications for living life as a man. As long as you meet over a cold beer or a rare steak, you don't have to call it a book club.

Mix a Specialty Cocktail... and Make Some Memories

YEARS AGO I was passing through Hamburg, Germany when a friend of a friend graciously opened his home and hosted me during my stay. I'll never forget Matthias's hospitality — a welcome respite amidst weeks of impersonal hotels and the solitude of solo travel. He went to great lengths to ensure that I, a complete stranger, received a full and rich experience of his city. He showed me the sights, introduced me to his favorite hidden gems, and gave me my first taste of the unexpectedly delicious German delicacy of currywurst (sliced bratwurst smothered in curried ketchup).

On my second night in town, Matthias organized a dinner party to introduce me to his friends. While I'm sure the company was great and the food delicious, over time the faces and tastes of that night have faded into distant memory. There is, however, one element that I can still recall with perfect clarity. My enduring memory of that night is the specialty cocktail that was served — Bombay Crushed. Somehow the cocktail immediately broke the ice and soon an American stranger felt at complete ease amongst instant German friends. For me, the sweet refreshment of Bombay Crushed will forever be linked with warm spring nights, lively, dynamic conversation, relaxed fun, and new friendships.

A few years later, as I planned my wedding, strong memories of my time in Hamburg came vividly flooding back. I fondly remembered the inexplicable way in which a special yet simple drink seemingly broke down barriers, facilitating great conversation and fellowship among strangers. So, on a beautiful, picturesque July day on Martha's Vineyard, two handpicked specialty cocktails were served, setting the tone for the event's relaxed New England island charm. Looking back on our wedding day, my wife and I will always cherish how smoothly and comfortably different groups of friends and family integrated together, rising above the ease and safety of their inherent cliques. Sure, there were other more important factors at play that day but I'll be forever thankful to our bartender nonetheless!

In many ways, living a life more gentlemanly is about developing meaningful relationships and enriching the lives of others. At first blush it may seem silly, but I've found that special cocktails have a special way of heightening special occasions. I have many dear memories indelibly linked to a specific drink: slinging back Singapore Slings at their iconic birthplace, the Raffles Hotel Long Bar; my martini inauguration

Signature Mocktails

Do you or your guests abstain from alcohol? Find a nonalcoholic recipe; as long as the drink is unique and unexpected, it will be welcomed with enthusiasm and remembered with fondness. Here are some examples:

HORSE'S NECK
Peel the whole rind of a lemon, in one spiraling piece. Place it in a tumbler with one end hanging over the top. Add two cubes of ice and a dash of bitters, then fill the tumbler with ginger ale.

PUSSYFOOT
Combine two ounces orange juice, two ounces lemon juice, one ounce lime juice, one teaspoon grenadine, and one egg yolk in a cocktail shaker and shake well over ice. Strain into an old-fashioned glass filled with ice cubes.

NOT SO DARK AND STORMY
In a wide mouthed glass, combine ice, $1/4$ cup of fresh lime juice, and $1/2$ tsp molasses. Add I cup of ginger beer. Stir well, until molasses has dissolved. Garnish with a lime wedge.

(extra-dry, gin, with a twist) as a new NYC ad agency exec with one of the old guard at a hidden speakeasy; and bottomless Bahama Mamas — a lethally smooth concoction of rum and fresh fruit juices — mixed on a small deserted Caribbean island. I'm sure you have your own fond recollections of good times with good drink. Let's make more memories!

SELECTION: CONSIDER SEASON, SCENE, AND THEME
How do you choose from thousands of cocktail recipes?

Consider the season. One thing that can make signature cocktails so distinctive is the use of whole fruit, fresh fruit juice, or fruit purées. The Bombay Crushed, for which I have so much nostalgia, was memorable in large part due to the perfect ripeness of the in-season kumquats. Recipes that utilize seasonal fruit often match the feel of the season in flavor and consistency, so think about what's in season and look for a recipe that takes advantage of the freshest fruit available at your local market.

Another consideration for cocktail selection is the scene. Scotch is always more at home in a wood-paneled library than on a bright, sunny beach. Dark liquor is generally more flavorful and feels heavier than light liquor so it's better suited for nighttime events. If you choose to use darker liquor for a daytime event, make sure to brighten it up with something like mint as in the case of mint juleps. Rum instantly injects a summery, Caribbean feel into a cocktail. Warm-weather outdoor events call for fresh and light mixtures, while dark, hearty, spicy cocktails can warm up the coldest of nights. As you read ingredient lists, trust your gut instinct, and don't underestimate a name — if a drink sounds out of place in your event's setting, it probably is.

If your event has a theme, you might want to carry it through to your cocktail. Serve mai tais at a luau, spiced cider at a Halloween party, or eggnog at a holiday event. If you're throwing a party for a Brazilian friend, serve caipirinhas. Color can be another fun way to distinguish your cocktail and tie it into an event. Liquors like blue curaçao (pronounced "cure-a-sow," as in curing a female pig) can add a dynamic punch of color to your bash. My wife and I recently threw a baby gender reveal party and the pink and blue cocktails were a huge hit.

Finally, experiment and have fun. The most signature of signature cocktails is the one you create on your own.

BOMBAY CRUSHED

4 kumquats

2 ounces simple syrup (or 2 teaspoons brown sugar)

$1/3$ ounce lime juice

Crushed ice

6 ounces Bombay Sapphire Gin

Halve the kumquats and place them in a glass. Add the simple syrup or brown sugar and lime juice. Lightly crush the kumquats with a pestle. Fill the glass with crushed ice and add the Bombay. Stir with a bar spoon and serve immediately.

CAIPIRINHA

2 teaspoons superfine sugar

I lime, cut into eight wedges

Ice cubes

2 $1/2$ ounces cachaça

Muddle the sugar and lime wedges in an old-fashioned glass. Fill glass with ice cubes and add the cachaça. Stir well.

BLUE LAGOON

I $1/2$ ounces blue curaçao

I $1/2$ ounces vodka

Ice cubes

6 ounces lemonade

I cherry or lime wedge

Pour the blue curaçao and vodka over ice cubes. Add the lemonade and stir. Garnish with cherry or lime wedge.

MIX A SPECIALTY COCKTAIL...
AND MAKE SOME MEMORIES

11

QUESTION TO CONTEMPLATE When you think back on fond memories, what details endure? Is there any consistency to the details that you remember across events? Is it possible for us to create stronger, longer-lasting memories in the present?

GENTLEMANLY QUOTE TO REMEMBER "There cannot be good living where there is not good drinking."

— Benjamin Franklin

ACTION STEP Find an excuse to serve a specialty cocktail and make some memories! Experiment with drink recipes and then host a dinner or cocktail party, break the mold at your next poker night, or impress on your next date night.

From Dandy to Handy: Emergency Car Care

WHEN MY PARENTS GOT MARRIED, they were still students on a budget, so my father had to learn how to fix everything himself. If the faucet was dripping, they weren't sleeping. If the washing machine broke, they were scrubbing clothes in the bathtub. Perhaps most dauntingly, if the car wasn't running, they were walking. This experience, coupled with a PhD in mechanical engineering, means that today my father can take apart a car and put it back together with not much more than a screwdriver and a kitchen fork. Over the years, my father's DIY approach to problem-solving has resulted in more than a few humorous home remedies, but when I need fix-it advice, there's no doubt whom I call first.

However, despite my father's best attempts to pass along his knowledge, I struggle installing a window air conditioner (and in one of my least handy moments, I once lowered a car too quickly, pinning my dad's thumb between the car and jack . . . ouch! Sorry, Dad.)

If you, like me, worry that your mechanical shortcomings might leave you stranded on the side of the road one day, this chapter is for you.

CHANGING A CAR TIRE

Perhaps no other handy task is more romanticized than changing a car tire. Admit it, you've daydreamed about being the hero who saves the roadside damsel in distress. Make sure you're ready for your knight-in-shining armor moment with these step-by-step instructions.

YOU WILL NEED: lug wrench, car jack, spare tire

I. SAFETY FIRST. Take stock of your surroundings; you want to be on solid, level ground, as far from traffic as possible. It is always preferable to slowly drive a short distance on a flat tire than change it in a dangerous or exposed location. Place the vehicle in park for an automatic transmission or reverse for a manual transmission. Place a wheel chock (or brick/large rock) diagonally opposite the wheel being changed to keep the car from rolling once you jack it up. Remove the ignition key, engage the emergency brake, and turn on the hazard lights before getting started.

2. NUT CRACKER. This is where all that gym time pays off. Remove the hubcap to expose the lug nuts, if necessary, and

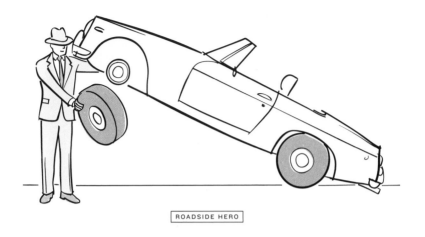

ROADSIDE HERO

use the lug wrench to loosen them by turning counterclockwise. (Some lugs have left-handed threads, usually identified with a stamped "L" on the lug bolt. In this case, turn clockwise.) Find you've been putting in more time on the couch than in the gym? Place the lug wrench on the nut so that it is horizontal with the ground and stand/stomp on it. Still struggling? Spray a little WD-40 on the lug nuts and let it sit for a few minutes. Crack the lug nuts loose but don't remove them at this point.

3. GET JACKED. Check for the correct placement of the jack in the owner's manual. If you find yourself on less-than-solid ground, use a piece of plywood as your base. Crank the jack up until the wheel is clear of the ground.

4. FREEWHEELIN'. Remove the loosened lug nuts by hand and take off the flat tire. Replace the flat with the spare, tightening the lug nuts back into place as far as possible by hand.

5. TIGHTEN UP. Lower the jack until the wheel just touches the ground. Tighten the lug nuts with the wrench following this pattern:

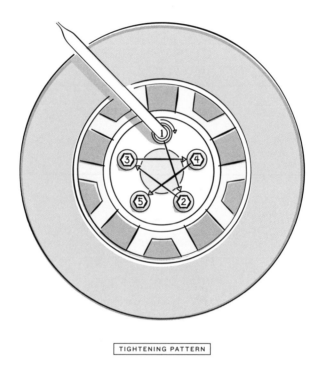

TIGHTENING PATTERN

Lower the jack all the way and give the lug nuts another tightening. After a few miles, pull over and give the lugs one final tightening.

YOU WILL NEED: a car with a charged battery, jumper cables

Is there anything more emasculating than calling roadside service for a simple flat battery? Save yourself from an embarrassing phone call by learning the very simple steps for jump-starting a car.

1. Turn off both cars.
2. Connect one of the cable's **red** clamps to the **positive** terminal of the **flat battery.**
3. Connect the other **red** clamp to the positive terminal of the **good battery.**
4. Connect a **black** clamp to the negative terminal of the **good battery.**
5. Ground the other **black** clamp by connecting it to a clean metal surface somewhere under the hood of the stalled car. DO NOT connect the second black clamp to the battery.
6. Start the car with the good battery and let it run for two or three minutes. Then start the car with the flat battery.
7. Remove the cables in the reverse order that they were placed. Be careful to avoid fan blades and belts of the running engines.
8. Stand back and congratulate yourself for saving the time and dignity waiting for service assistance would have killed.

12   FROM DANDY TO HANDY: EMERGENCY CAR RESCUE

QUESTION TO CONTEMPLATE If being a man means being dependable, do you have the knowledge and skills to step in when needed?

GENTLEMANLY QUOTE TO REMEMBER "One only needs two tools in life: WD-40 to make things go, and duct tape to make them stop."

—G.M. Weilacher

ACTION STEP Practice changing a tire in your driveway so that you can familiarize yourself with the process for your car in a safe environment. You don't want your first attempt to be while wearing a suit, late on your way to the airport, at night, in the rain, on the side of a major freeway, do you?

Why the Tie Should Never Die

THE MODERN NECKTIE has been on a steady decline since its popularity peaked in 1995. A casualty of the dot-com era and its casual workplace mentality, this bastion of masculinity is finally falling from favor. And this is precisely why the modern gentleman *should* wear a tie. Not just to keep some nostalgic item from becoming an artifact, but because men are simply better off with a tie knotted elegantly around their neck. Wear a tie because it makes you look good. Wear a tie because it makes you feel put-together. Wear a tie to stand out. Wear a tie because people will treat you differently when you wear it. Most of all, wear a tie because it's a sign of respect — for yourself, your job, and everyone you come in contact with.

In 1989, the Pratt knot was introduced on the front page of the *New York Times.* It was the first new tie knot to emerge in over fifty years. Unwilling to wait another half-century for another knot breakthrough, two research fellows at Cambridge University's Cavendish Laboratory applied mathematics to the cause and discovered that there are exactly eighty-five ways to tie a tie.

For all practical purposes, most of the eighty-five knots are novelties. In fact, the authors themselves deemed only thirteen of the eighty-five aesthetically pleasing enough for common usage. The modern man only needs to know three tie knots: one for daily use, one for fancy use, and one for super-fancy, or otherwise jaunty use.

FOR DAILY USE: THE FOUR-IN-HAND KNOT

The etymology of the four-in-hand knot is attributed to English four-in-hand carriage drivers who were said to either use the knot on their reins or their neck scarves. Regardless, today the four-in-hand is the most common tie knot in the world, and is the regulation tie knot for the United States Navy. Simple, elegant, and slightly asymmetrical, the four-in-hand is a versatile go-to knot for everyday use.

STEP 1: Cross the wide end over the narrow end.

STEP 2: Wrap the wide end beneath the narrow end.

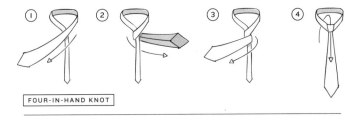

FOUR-IN-HAND KNOT

STEP 3: Bring the wide end back over the narrow end.

STEP 4: Pull the wide end up and through the back of the loop and then down through the loop to knot it.

FOR FANCY USE: THE WINDSOR KNOT

The Windsor knot results in a wide, triangular, symmetrical knot. Because of its girth, the Windsor is best for shirts with a cutaway or spread collar. Erroneously credited to the Duke of Windsor, the Windsor knot was more likely a creation of his father, George V. The knot's symmetry gives it an almost ceremonial presence best suited for formal events. The Windsor is the prescribed knot for the British Royal Air Force and its cadets, as well as all Canadian Armed Forces.

STEP 1: Start with the wide end hanging on the right side, much longer than the narrow end.

STEP 2: Cross the wide end over the narrow end and bring it up through the center hole.

STEP 3: Bring the wide end beneath the narrow end, and up

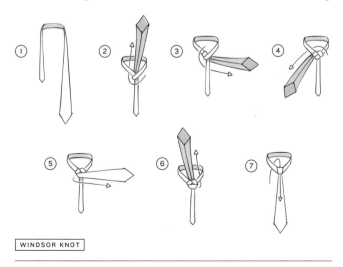

WINDSOR KNOT

towards the right side (the back of the wide end should now be facing up).

STEP 4: Put the wide end through the center hole, wrapping a loop around the right side of the tie (the wide end should still be facing upside down).

STEP 5: Cross the wide end over the whole knot.

STEP 6: Pull the wide end up through the loop.

STEP 7: Pass the wide end down, through the knot in front.

FOR SUPER-FANCY, OR OTHERWISE JAUNTY USE: THE BOW TIE

The bow tie is an interesting case study in split personality. On the one hand, the bow tie is the most formal of all neckwear, and the only suitable choice for black-tie or white-tie occasions. On the other hand, thanks to its wide availability in bold, fun fabrics, the bow tie is also a whimsical, contrarian, "devil-may-care" accessory for less formal use.

In whichever context you choose to wear the bow tie, learn to tie it properly. Pretied bow ties are for male strippers and bad rental tuxedos, not the neck of a gentleman. (A pretied bow tie is attached to its neckband by a metal clip or buckle, visible with a wing-collar shirt and a sure sign of tackiness for all to see.) A proper, self-tied bow tie requires slightly more effort to accomplish, but the upgrade in class, comfort, and elegance cannot be overstated.

> **"The manner in which a man ties his bow tie distinguishes a man of genius from a mediocre one."**
>
> **—HONORÉ BALZAC**

By virtue of its need to be tied, the self-tied bow tie is easier to fit comfortably than one that is pretied. The self-tied bow also allows for a slightly imperfect presentation, giving the wearer a certain stylish *je ne sais quoi* unachievable with the factory-tied bow.

Here's how to tie a bow tie like a genius:

STEP 1: Pass the right side over the left and under to form a simple knot.

STEP 2: Fold the right side into a bow shape with the narrowest part directly over your button.

STEP 3: Hang the loose end over the center of the bow.

STEP 4: There should now be a loop between the base knot and the front of the bow.

STEP 5: Pass the middle of the loose end of the bow behind the bow and through the loop.

STEP 6: Pull the loose end halfway through and tighten the bow by tugging on the two opposite loops.

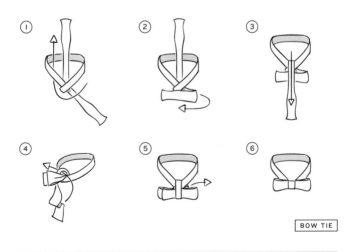

BOW TIE

13

WHY THE TIE SHOULD NEVER DIE

QUESTION TO CONTEMPLATE How do you feel when you wear a tie? How do others feel when you wear a tie?

GENTLEMANLY QUOTE TO REMEMBER "A well-tied tie is the first serious step in life."

— OSCAR WILDE

ACTION STEP Make your own statement by wearing a tie somewhere unexpected, be it to class or the office during the week, on a date Saturday night, or to church on Sunday. Take note of what other people say to you, and how they may treat you differently.

Personal Philosophy for
Practical Purpose

IN 523 AD, THE ROMAN philosopher
Boethius was at the height of his power as
magister officiorum, head of all government and
court services. However, the position also
made him a target, and through treachery
and betrayal, Boethius was charged by his
rivals with treason and sentenced to death.
In prison, falsely accused and awaiting exe-
cution, Boethius wrote *The Consolation of
Philosophy,* a conversation between himself
and the allegorical Lady Philosophy, who
comforts him in his despair. Lady Philosophy points out that Boethius has become too
attached to the things of this world, which
are fleeting, bestowed and snatched away by
the fickle vagaries of "the wheel of fortune."

Lady Philosophy proffers that man should focus therefore not on temporal things (honor, power, health, wealth), but on matters of the mind, which are immune to the vicissitudes of fortune. Boethius concludes that only if a man can cultivate and live with virtue can he ever realize true happiness and satisfaction.

Although it has fallen out of the modern masculine lexicon, virtue has always been at the core of what it means to be a man, and indeed, a gentleman. Virtue comes from the Latin *virtutem,* meaning "moral strength, manliness, valor, excellence, worth," which itself comes from *vir,* meaning "man."

BENJAMIN FRANKLIN'S THIRTEEN VIRTUES

Like Boethius, Benjamin Franklin valued the pursuit of virtue. At the age of twenty, Franklin embarked on a journey ambitious even for the man who would go on to become one of the most revered authors, scientists, inventors, and statesmen in American history — a quest for "moral perfection." Recognizing he would need all the help he could get to attempt such an audacious goal, Franklin set about developing a list of virtues to direct his life. He settled on thirteen:

1. TEMPERANCE. "Eat not to dullness; drink not to elevation."
2. SILENCE. "Speak not but what may benefit others or yourself; avoid trifling conversation."
3. ORDER. "Let all your things have their places; let each part of your business have its time."
4. RESOLUTION. "Resolve to perform what you ought; perform without fail what you resolve."
5. FRUGALITY. "Make no expense but to do good to others or yourself; i.e., waste nothing."

6. INDUSTRY. "Lose no time; be always employ'd in something useful; cut off all unnecessary actions."

7. SINCERITY. "Use no hurtful deceit; think innocently and justly, and, if you speak, speak accordingly."

8. JUSTICE. "Wrong none by doing injuries, or omitting the benefits that are your duty."

9. MODERATION. "Avoid extremes; forbear resenting injuries so much as you think they deserve."

10. CLEANLINESS. "Tolerate no uncleanliness in body, cloaths, or habitation."

11. TRANQUILITY. "Be not disturbed at trifles, or at accidents common or unavoidable."

12. CHASTITY. "Rarely use venery but for health or offspring, never to dullness, weakness, or the injury of your own or another's peace or reputation."

13. HUMILITY. "Imitate Jesus and Socrates."

Franklin carried around a checklist of his thirteen virtues, marking an X next to each virtue he failed to live up to each day. At the end of the week, he would review the list with the goal of achieving a clean sheet. Franklin never did succeed in his quest for moral perfection (beer and women were especially troublesome), but over time he did see fewer and fewer X marks and experience more and more personal happiness.

DEVELOP YOUR OWN PHILOSOPHY OF LIFE

Franklin presents a compelling example to the modern gentleman for creating a personal philosophy of life. A personal philosophy is an articulated and documented collection of your ideas and beliefs about how the world works and your role in it. A written philosophy provides the gentleman with a firm and defensible foundation upon which to base decisions and opinions. Without one, the gentleman is not strongly rooted, and more susceptible to the uncontrollable machinations of Boethius's "wheel of fortune." And only through this articulation can a gentleman examine, correct, or embrace his beliefs as required.

Ready to get started? Begin with the statement, "I believe . . ." and make a list of things that you believe, hold true, or find self-evident. Don't be too overcautious on your first run-through; step two is culling the list down. After finishing your first draft, review the list and remove anything that seems inconsequential or repetitive, and start combining the remaining belief statements into logical groups. Come up with a new statement that accurately and collectively summarizes each group. In this way you should end up with a list of no more than ten strong, meaningful beliefs.

Asking hard, self-reflective questions can really help the "I believe . . ." exercise. Here are some questions that I find particularly useful:

- What directs my actions and decisions, especially the impulsive ones?

- What gives me a sense of satisfaction?

- On my current trajectory, where am I headed? Do I want to go there?

- What do I want my legacy to be?

- What do I value more than anything in theory?

- What do I value most in actual practice? Is there a consistent struggle in my life?

- How did I spend my free time this past week?

- What most excites me?

- What most scares me?

- What am I most proud of?

- What am I most grateful for?

- What is my ideal day?

- What is my purpose in life?

- Why do I exist?

- What is my mission?

Another useful exercise in developing your own set of values is an examination of historical quotations. Some people have an amazing gift for eloquently and poignantly capturing their beliefs in succinct statements to which we can only react, "Yes!" I would suggest that you do this *after* working to create belief statements of your own, and to try to focus on the content of the quotation, rather than the authorship or wit with which it is delivered. Try creating a list of ten quotes that describe you and your philosophy of life. Compare it to your list of belief statements, and share your list with those who know you best as a check. If you're living life with integrity to your values, the list should be instantly recognizable to others as a genuine reflection of your character.

GO TO THE MOUNTAINTOP

We live in a time-starved, instant-gratification, media-saturated society. The world tells us we need to live in perpetual motion, overstuffing our schedules and craving constant stimulation. But as we strive to jam as many job promotions, awards, experiences, friendships, and activities into our lives as possible, we lose the ability to sit back and reflect on whether any of it really matters.

SELF-REFLECTION IS NECESSARY. Without it we're driving through life without a map, foot to the floor, hoping we'll ultimately arrive where we should. In order for values to be useful, they must be actively owned, not simply inherited. Too many of us take our values from our parents or a confident, charismatic friend; from the pulpit; or a talking head on TV. We accept what others believe as truth, without taking the time to consider important issues for ourselves.

SOLITUDE IS IMPORTANT. The modern world is so interconnected and constantly plugged in that finding the time and space to think can be difficult. However, without freedom from the influence and distractions of the world, it is virtually impossible to develop well-reasoned opinions, ideas, and values. History is littered with examples of the transcendent power of solitude. Darwin took long, solitary walks and emphatically turned down dinner party invitations. Moses spent time alone in the desert. Jesus wandered the wilderness. Mohammed sat in the cave. Buddha went to the mountaintop. Find your own mountaintop and don't come down without your own thoughts, opinions, and values.

14

PERSONAL PHILOSOPHY FOR PRACTICAL PURPOSE

QUESTION TO CONTEMPLATE What code of values and beliefs are you consciously or subconsciously living by? When you evaluate the code you live by, does it match the code you *want* to live by?

GENTLEMANLY QUOTE TO REMEMBER "The ultimate value of life depends upon awareness and the power of contemplation rather than upon mere survival."

— Aristotle

ACTION STEP Go to the mountaintop. Intentionally set aside time for self-reflection — perhaps fifteen minutes every morning, an hour per week, or a full day every quarter. Seek the solitude to evaluate *what* you believe and *why.* Develop an ownable set of values on which you can build a life free from the machinations of the "wheel of fortune" and consistently evaluate your actions, thoughts, and decisions against your values.

Well Packed: Inside a Gentleman's Travel Bag

THE ENGLISH WORD FOR "TRAVEL" originates from the medieval French word "travail," meaning suffering, painful effort, or trouble. While travel is easier and faster than it was in the Middle Ages, obtrusive security procedures, long lines, overcrowding, excessive fees, and seemingly inexplicable delays can certainly make modern travel seem painful. While there's not much the modern gentleman can do about crying babies or overzealous security agents, one thing within his control is what and how he packs, to ensure he's ready for any situation, even when miles away from home.

THE PACK MENTALITY

Keep these qualities in mind when packing items for your trip.

VERSATILE. Perhaps the most important characteristic for anything you pack is its versatility. Prioritize items that play well with others and can be dressed up and down.

LIGHTWEIGHT. Heavy items add bulk to your load, and can crush less-substantial packed items (like dress shirts). Opt for multiple, lighter layers rather than heavy outerwear. Leather jackets, overcoats, and boots are best left at home or, if required, worn while traveling.

LOW MAINTENANCE. Even in nice hotels, poorly maintained in-room irons can be dangerous to fine cotton, and finding a quality dry cleaner is risky enough at home; on the road it's an absolute crapshoot. Leave high-maintenance fabrics like linen at home and opt for less fussy materials like denim and wool.

SEVEN TRAVEL MUST-HAVES

A NAVY BLAZER. Because it's formal enough to class up jeans for a night out, and informal enough to use as an extra layer around town if the temperature dips. The navy blazer once again proves its worth as the most versatile item in a man's closet (and suitcase).

V-NECK SWEATER. Because planes are notoriously cold, and even in warm climates, nights can get cool. A lightweight V-neck is versatile (wear it under a suit or with jeans) and stylish, making it the ideal layering tool for travel.

A DARK, SOLID SUIT. Because if you need a suit for work, this one can pull double duty. Dark, solid-colored suit jackets and pants can be worn as separates just as successfully as together. Lose the tie, swap your suit pants for jeans, and you're ready to go from boardroom to taproom.

NON-IRON SHIRTS. Because ironing on the road is a pain. Normally I don't recommend wrinkle-resistant shirts, which can feel a bit stiff and rough, but when traveling I make an exception. However, if you've got sensitive skin, the trade-off between convenience and comfort might not be worth it.

SOMETHING TO READ. Because you need an escape from transit waiting times and overly chatty, yet dull, seatmates. View the downtime as an opportunity to read something you especially enjoy, or have been meaning to get around to.

A PREPACKED DOPP KIT. Because otherwise you're ensured a frenzied, last-minute bathroom scramble. Prepack your kit with travel-sized toiletry duplicates or you might return home without your only stick of deodorant.

EXTRA UNDERWEAR. Because impromptu travel changes happen and, while you can rewear most other clothes, a gentleman always wears clean underwear.

WHAT NOT TO PACK

FRENCH CUFF SHIRTS. Unless you plan on wearing a dinner jacket, leave the double cuffs and corresponding easy-to-misplace cufflinks at home.

YOUR LAPTOP. In an age of smartphones and tablets, if you're not traveling for business there's really no need for the extra weight and security screening hassle of a laptop. Prioritize the people and places you're visiting by leaving the temptation of work behind.

ANYTHING YOU CAN BUY OR RENT INEXPENSIVELY AT YOUR DESTINATION. On a trip to Hawaii, I once packed my own snorkeling gear. When we arrived I was kicking myself for taking up so much room in my bag once I realized the hotel rented the same gear at very reasonable rates.

ANYTHING PACKED WHILE SAYING "WHAT IF . . ." Chances are good you won't need it.

FOLD YOUR SUIT JACKET WITH MERCY

STEP 1: Lay the jacket facedown, with the back facing you.
STEP 2: Invert the right-side shoulder so that it is inside out.
STEP 3: Fold the left side of the jacket along the back centerline.

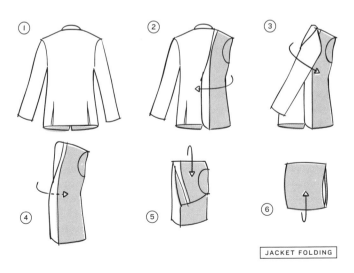

JACKET FOLDING

STEP 4: Nestle the left shoulder inside of the inside-out right shoulder to protect against crush damage.

STEP 5: Fold the jacket in half or thirds, depending on the width of your bag.

STEP 6: Step back and congratulate yourself on protecting your sartorial investment.

PACKING TIPS

• Folding clothing with a plastic bag or tissue paper sandwiched between layers can reduce the friction and crumpling that cause wrinkles.

• Before a trip, ask your dry cleaner to fold your shirts instead of hang them. The perfectly folded, consistently shaped rectangles are ready-made for your suitcase.

• Rolling clothes like T-shirts and underwear can be a valuable space saver.

• If you don't have a tie case, protect your tie by wrapping it around a toilet paper roll and placing it into a small sealable plastic bag.

• Always place shoes and other heavy items at the bottom of your bag to prevent them from crushing other items.

• The bundle technique efficiently utilizes space and reduces wrinkling. The technique involves wrapping clothing in concentric layers around a core, resulting in a large bundle. A jacket or suit, folded as suggested in this chapter, makes a great core, as does a T-shirt wrapped around socks and underwear. Start with the most wrinkle-resistant clothing first, and alternate collars and waistbands to ensure an even shape.

WELL PACKED: INSIDE A GENTLEMAN'S TRAVEL BAG

QUESTION TO CONTEMPLATE How does being well-packed impact a trip? Do you pack with care and intention or haphazardly on your way out the door? Does it matter?

GENTLEMANLY QUOTE TO REMEMBER "He who would travel happily must travel light."
— Antoine de Saint-Exupéry

ACTION STEP Practice the folding techniques outlined in this chapter. Use them on your next trip.

The Courage to Encourage

WALT WHITMAN is a giant of modern literature, yet for many years he struggled as nothing more than an aspiring writer. In the midst of his discouragement, Whitman received a letter of affirmation: "Dear Sir, I am not blind to the worth of the wonderful gift of *Leaves of Grass*. I find it the most extraordinary piece of wit and wisdom that America has yet contributed. I am very happy in reading it, as great power makes us happy...I greet you at the beginning of a great career." The letter was signed Ralph Waldo Emerson. Of course, Whitman went on to have a long and successful career, but without the encouragement of his literary idol, perhaps his life would have taken a different course.

Encouragement is powerful. It's rocket fuel for the journey of life, propelling us upward against the gravitational pull of mediocrity and adversity, and toward the heavenly possibilities of who we can, and should, become. Study after study has shown a clear link between encouragement and everything from child development and growth to increased physical performance and professional advancement. Encouragement gives us the courage we need to become more than we are — to take risks, persevere, stretch to reach goals, and stand firm on our principles.

EVEN THE PRESIDENT NEEDS ENCOURAGEMENT

On display at the Library of Congress in Washington, D.C. are the contents of Abraham Lincoln's pockets from the night of his assassination. The eyeglasses, pocketknife, and other everyday articles paint a very human picture of the man that history has elevated to near mythological status. Perhaps most telling is an old newspaper clipping Lincoln carried in his wallet, praising his presidency and referring to him as "one of the greatest statesmen of all time." Lincoln battled self-doubt, especially during the Civil War when criticism rained in from all sides. That even a man of Lincoln's stature should require a constant reminder of encouragement speaks to the absolutely universal human need for affirmation.

No matter what your station in life, there are people within your immediate sphere of influence who need your encouragement. As a father or husband, own the responsibility to encourage your family. As an organizational leader, boost the effectiveness of your team by championing and empowering the people you lead. Use the privilege of friendship to speak up and help transform your friends' lives. As American business man and philanthropist Truett Cathy, puts it, "How do you identify someone who needs encouragement? That person is breathing."

KEYS TO ENCOURAGEMENT

I have a friend whose young son plays soccer. The league doesn't keep score or even track winners and losers. At the end of the season, everybody gets a trophy, and presumably, no one's feelings are hurt.

In order for encouragement to be meaningful it must be genuine, specific, and warranted. Praise for praise's sake rings hollow, like a soccer trophy every kid gets—received, but not really earned. True encouragement is more than coddling or

---

ENCOURAGEMENT MULTIPLIERS

The impact of your encouragement can be amplified when it is:

UNEXPECTED. Offering encouragement to someone for something that might easily go unnoticed is your way of signaling you truly care.

PUBLIC. Encouragement given in front of other people is all the more affirming because it shows the conviction behind your words.

SUPPORTED WITH ACTION. You can cheer someone on, or you can cheer someone on and then give a helping hand. Combine your encouragement with a beneficial introduction, a helpful favor, or useful gift.

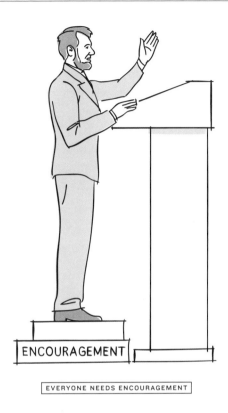

ENCOURAGEMENT

EVERYONE NEEDS ENCOURAGEMENT

ego stroking, it is purpose-driven. Here's how to ensure your encouragement is the real deal:

SHOW GENUINE INTEREST As the saying goes, "Nobody cares how much you know until they know how much you care." Ask questions and listen enthusiastically. Only after you know someone's story can you adequately impact it.

ADDRESS PSYCHOLOGICAL NEEDS As humans, we all crave fulfillment of certain psychological needs. Psychologist Abraham Maslow famously described these as self-actualization and esteem in his hierarchy of needs. We all want to feel part of something larger than ourselves. We all want to solve problems and improve things that need improving. We all want to feel respected and valued by others. We all want to be proud of what we've accomplished. The best encouragement will address, at least in part, one or more of these needs.

MAKE YOUR ENCOURAGEMENT ACTIONABLE Compliments are nice to hear, but encouragement can be so much more. If you intend for your words to result in action, frame them that way. "That's such an innovative and fresh way of approaching this problem. I think you're really onto something. Start with XYZ and let me know if I can help!"

ENCOURAGEMENT DOES NOT REQUIRE AGREEMENT

It's easy to offer encouragement in situations where you agree with what someone is doing. Encouragement comes a bit harder when a friend or family member has decided to do something you don't agree with. If the person's mind is made up, even after you've voiced your concern, you may be tempted to wash your hands of the whole thing. After all, if the person isn't going to listen to you, why should you stick around, right? Wrong.

Weigh your own emotional response to the situation. Are you projecting your own experiences or feelings onto someone else's life? If your brother wants to quit his job and become a rodeo clown, you may think it's a poor decision based on your own experience as a rodeo clown. However, the reality is that your brother's experience may not mirror your own, and perhaps your encouragement might make the difference. Also consider that the things we are most vocal about are often the things we ourselves fear the most. At the end of the day you aren't the judge and jury for what should or shouldn't make someone happy. Unless someone's decision will directly harm him or herself or others, withholding encouragement and support is never the gentlemanly thing to do.

A NEW KIND OF ACCOUNTABILITY

I meet with a group of men every Thursday morning in the SoHo neighborhood of Manhattan. Getting up before the sun rises is never easy, but on Thursday mornings, five A.M. can't come soon enough. I often tell people that Thursday mornings have completely transformed my life. There isn't much of a formal agenda, but one of our stated missions is to encourage one another and keep each other accountable, not to the things we shouldn't be doing, but rather to the things we should be doing — the passions and dreams that are in our hearts. There's already enough accountability for making mistakes in the world. When we mess up, we hear all about it, and frankly, it's not always very helpful. By comparison, it's so refreshing to give and receive accountability that focuses on potential, not problems. It's a new kind of accountability, and for me it has made all the difference.

THE COURAGE TO ENCOURAGE

QUESTION TO CONTEMPLATE People generally fall into one of three (nonexclusive) categories: the Naysayer, who rains on parades; the Islander, who might mean well, but is often too self-absorbed to notice or help others; and the Booster, who enhances the lives of others by championing and inspiring them to become better versions of themselves. Everyone who comes in contact with a booster is enriched and empowered by the experience. What kind of person are you? What kind of person do you want to be?

GENTLEMANLY QUOTE TO REMEMBER "Treat a man as he appears to be and you make him worse. But treat a man as if he already were what he potentially could be, and you make him what he should be."
— JOHANN GOETHE

ACTION STEP Encouragement costs nothing to give, yet can mean everything to receive. Think of a close friend or family member who could use some encouragement. Commit to call that person in the next three days. Meanwhile, intentionally look out for an opportunity to encourage someone today, even a complete stranger. Be brave!

Deliver a Toast Worth Drinking To

IT'S AN ENJOYABLE (even if probably untrue) bit of folk wisdom that our tradition of clinking glasses originated from a time when the fear of being poisoned was so great that glasses were knocked together in order to spill over and mix the contents of drinks. While the chances of someone slipping hemlock into your champagne might be slim these days, toasts still strike fear in the hearts of men. For some of our gender, public speaking can cause more angst than receding hairlines, impotence, and stock portfolio plummets combined. Here's how to confidently and articulately deliver a toast that won't tempt you, or the rest of the room, to reintroduce the poison.

On a cold, wet day in 1841, William Henry Harrison gave the longest inaugural speech in U.S. history. The 8,445-word speech exposed the hatless and coatless president to the unforgiving elements for hours. Three weeks later he was dead from

---

THE GLOBETROTTER TOASTER

Want to clink glasses overseas without causing an international incident? Brush up on local customs and etiquette.

- CHINA: *Baijiu* is commonly hailed as the national drink of China, and if you ever find yourself at a family celebration or business negotiation, you'll be drinking a lot of it. Touching another person's glass below the rim is a sign of honor and respect.

- JAPAN: When in Japan, the honored guest should always offer a *kanpai* (meaning "bottoms up" or "dry glass") shortly after the host or at the conclusion of the meal.

- GERMANY: When toasting, declare *Prost!* ("cheers") with beer or *Zum Wohl!* ("good health") when drinking wine. Maintain eye contact from the time the glass is lifted until it is placed back on the table or else you're doomed to seven years of bad sex!

- RUSSIA: Don't eat or drink anything until the host has made the first toast. The second toast should follow quickly or as the Cossack expression goes, "Between the first and second toasts, a bullet should not pass." Always finish your drink before placing your glass back on the table.

- ISRAEL: It is acceptable to just touch the glass to your lips if you don't wish to drink after the typical toast *L'chaim* ("to life").

pneumonia and pleurisy. The lesson? Don't talk yourself to death! Nothing will doom a toast more assuredly than long-winded rambling. Keep your toast direct and to the point or risk losing the room. Remember, when people tune out and aren't focused on you, more consequentially, they aren't focused on the subject of your toast either. At a formal event, try to limit your toast to between two and five minutes.

PRACTICE (AND SOBRIETY) MAKE PERFECT

Like other regrettable yet avoidable aspects of life, two things can prevent rambling: preparation and sobriety. Public speaking experts claim that great preparation reduces anxiety and fear by 70 to 80 percent. As a general rule, plan to apply one hour of prep time per minute of speaking time. Practice will also ensure you can deliver your toast without notes and save you from the decidedly non-suave notecard and drink juggling act. That pregame slug might seem like a confidence booster but Jack Daniel's and Johnnie Walker are more likely to hijack your words than help them. Save the alcohol for after the "hip, hip, hoorays."

WORDSMITH FOR SUCCESS

Your words should be kind and gracious; this is not the time for a roast. Keep things personal but avoid inside jokes or stories that no one else will understand. Remember the point of your toast is to celebrate someone else, so keep the focus firmly on him or her. A common mistake is talking about yourself too much instead of the person you're making the toast to. Personal stories and anecdotes can add context but any more than a little can make a genuine gesture seem self-serving quickly. Avoid embarrassing topics, ex-wives, or old boyfriends, and never force comedy. Either you're funny or you're not; if you aren't sure which applies to you, chances are it's the latter.

STEP UP AND SPEAK OUT

The moment of truth has arrived. Rise up to meet it with boldness and confidence like the man you want to be. Stand and wait for the room to quiet down. Standing should be enough, but if not, speak up with a polite but firm "Excuse me" or "May I have your attention, please." Don't rap your glass with silverware; it's uncouth, and broken Baccarat never gets a toast off on the right foot. While speaking, hold your drink up; it's not only appropriate but will give your hands something to do with all their nervous energy. (If your arm starts to get tired, that's a pretty good cue to wrap things up . . . or to start going back to the gym.) Speak slowly and clearly so everybody can hear you. Establish warmth by making eye contact, not only with the people you are giving the toast to but also everyone else in the room. However, make sure to end your toast looking at the person or people you are toasting.

AN EVERYDAY TOAST CAN MEAN THE MOST

Don't reserve your toasting talents just for weddings or other special occasions. The unexpected toast is often the most genuine and appreciated precisely because it's unexpected. Plus, the more toasts you give, the more comfortable you'll feel when that special event does come around. Toast to friends old and new. Toast to life lived to the full. Toast to love gained and lost. Toast to the beauty of art and the mystery of adventure. Toast to success or toast to adversity. It doesn't really matter what you toast, just that you raise your glass to something more than your lips.

If you're having trouble getting started, try this simple two-part formula: first, state the subject of your toast; then explain why it's worth toasting or offer well wishes on its behalf. For example: "To art—that which distinguishes man from beast." Or, "To Peter—may this new season of life bring excitement, joy, and fulfillment."

If your own words fail you, look for inspiration from the many legendary men who have raised a glass or two before us. In some situations a great quote alone might even suffice. Here are a few choice selections:

"With malice toward none; with charity for all."
— Abraham Lincoln

"May you live all the days of your life."
— Jonathan Swift

"A day for toil, an hour for sport. But for a friend life is too short."
— Ralph Waldo Emerson

"Fire is the test of gold; adversity of strong men."
— Seneca the Younger

"Without art, the crudeness of reality would make the world unbearable."
— George Bernard Shaw

"Who loves not women, wine, and song, remains a fool his whole life long."
— Martin Luther

"Come gentlemen, I hope we shall drink down all unkindness."
— William Shakespeare

DELIVER A TOAST WORTH DRINKING TO

 QUESTION TO CONTEMPLATE Who or what in your life is worth toasting? Are your feelings of gratitude or well wishes worth stepping out of your comfort zone to express, or will you let a simple fear keep you from honoring and celebrating those close to you?

 GENTLEMANLY QUOTE TO REMEMBER "Here's to us that are here, to you that are there, and the rest of us everywhere."

— Rudyard Kipling

 ACTION STEP A gentleman understands that a meaningful and well-articulated toast can take any event from ordinary to memorable. Don't wait for a wedding or state dinner to revive the informal yet thoughtful toasting tradition. Think about someone or something worth acknowledging and find an excuse to offer a toast at your next happy hour, dinner party, or even family night in. Better yet, keep the good times flowing by getting everyone to join you in proffering a toast or two of their own.

A Classical (Music) Education

You may think of classical music as outdated, and no more relevant to the modern gentleman than other vestiges of a bygone past like the top hat or a Latin education. However, what if you heard that classical music has been credited with aiding the maze navigation skills of lab rats, boosting the milk production of dairy cows, and increasing the intelligence of in utero babies, and that a German sewage treatment center even pipes Mozart into its plant to increase the efficacy of waste-consuming microbes, to save a thousand euros per month? Now, if classical music can give you an infallible sense of direction, an infinite supply of milk, genius-level intellect, and cash in your pocket, are you sure it's not for you?

Dubious mental and developmental benefits aside, what is undeniable is that classical music contains a level of nuance and depth that is very difficult to find on today's *Billboard* charts. Like anything of great value, full appreciation of classical music requires an investment of time and effort. Your investment won't go unrewarded, however; classical music gets better and richer the more you listen to it. Given the chance, the right piece can transcend mere notes and deliver the very essence of what it means to be human. So, even if you'd prefer more Boss than Beethoven on your iPod, it's important for today's well-rounded gentleman to have at least a cursory appreciation for classical music, whether for quiet contemplation, conversing with a music-loving client, or cramming for the GMAT.

Many find their first encounter with classical music confusing and intimidating. What follows is a highly subjective list, intended merely as an accessible jumping-off point for the amateur listener. Organized into three key eras of classical music, the list includes musical selections as well as compositional recommendations. While some choices may seem obvious to the more experienced listener, the list is intended as a helpful introduction for the beginner.

BAROQUE PERIOD (1600–1750)

Baroque music, like Baroque architecture, is characterized by elaborate ornamentation. In the same way that a Baroque church's facade has innumerable spires, curves, and carvings, baroque music contains multiple intricate melodies that intertwine, layer, and pass back and forth. Often described as the most cerebral of classical music, Baroque music is sophisticated and complex—the thinking man's choice.

THE BRANDENBURG CONCERTOS
JOHANN SEBASTIAN BACH

Bach is the most celebrated of the Baroque composers, and his Brandenburg Concertos exhibit the technical precision and sophistication for which he is so highly regarded. I'm especially partial to the 2005 recording by the Orchestra of the Age of Enlightenment.

WATER MUSIC
GEORGE FREDERIC HANDEL

Water Music contains three suites of celebratory airs and dances written for King George I and performed during a royal barge trip down the River Thames in 1717. An elegant, regal, and more leisurely counterpoint to Bach's more complex work. The 2001 recording by John Eliot Gardiner and the English Baroque Soloists is highly recommended.

THE GOLDBERG VARIATIONS
JOHANN SEBASTIAN BACH

Definitively recorded by Glenn Gould, first in 1955 and again in 1981, this sublime keyboard collection consists of an aria followed by thirty variations. Named for Johann Gottlieb Goldberg, their supposed first performer, *The Goldberg Variations* were originally subtitled by Bach ". . . for music lovers, to refresh their spirits," a feat they still accomplish to this day.

CLASSICAL PERIOD (1750–1800)

The difference between capital "C" Classical music (the specific era) and lowercase "c" classical music (the general umbrella term) is a point of confusion for many. The capitalized Classical era refers to a fifty-year period in which music

A Night at the Orchestra

For the philharmonic first-timer, the rituals and etiquette of the orchestra can be confusing. Here's what to expect:

• Most orchestras have (sadly) embraced the casual-ization of modern attire. Today's concert hall is filled with everything from jeans and T-shirts to three-piece suits (full black-tie regalia is a rarity except on opening night or other special gala events). However, you should buck the downward trend by wearing a suit. Your more formal attire will heighten the experience and is a nod of respect to the performers and venue.

• Arrive on time, which means at least fifteen to thirty minutes early. If you arrive after the performance has started you won't be seated until a break in the performance, if at all.

• The leader of the violin section is called the concertmaster. When the performance is about to begin, the concertmaster will walk onto the stage, the audience will applaud, and the concertmaster will bow. The concertmaster will then turn to the orchestra, a tuning note will sound, and the orchestra will tune itself. Next the conductor will appear on stage to more applause, shake hands with the concertmaster, and then turn to the orchestra. At this point the performance will begin.

• It's a major faux pas to applaud between movements. Use your program to keep track of the movements or wait for the conductor to lower his arms and turn to face the audience, your cue that the piece is finished. If all else fails, the safest option is to wait and follow the crowd's lead.

• Obviously, there should be no use of cell phones, eating, or drinking in the concert hall. If you have a cough, bring a supply of pre-unwrapped cough drops. If your cough persists, quietly excuse yourself from the hall until it is under control.

evolved to value simplicity over complexity. The Classical "homophonic" sound (single melody over supporting harmony) contrasts the "polyphonic" sound (multiple melodies layered over one another) of the Baroque period. The Classical era also saw movement towards heightened emotionalism, although not to the full extent of the ensuing Romantic period.

EINE KLEINE NACHTMUSIK
WOLFGANG AMADEUS MOZART
Perhaps the most easily recognizable and accessible of Mozart's work: infectious, elegant, and fun. Look for the fantastic 1985 recording by the Academy of St. Martin-in-the-Fields, conducted by Sir Neville Marriner.

SYMPHONY NO. 40
WOLFGANG AMADEUS MOZART
Along with the Twenty-fifth and Forty-first Symphonies, Symphony no. 40 is considered one of Mozart's finest. The first movement is a masterpiece of powerful restraint that some describe as a subtle expression of Mozart's increasingly hard life circumstances. Symphony no. 40 paved the way for more emotionally expressive and overtly powerful symphonies by Beethoven (who had great respect for no. 40) and the transition into the Romantic Period. The 1996 recording by Karl Bohm and the Berlin Philharmonic Orchestra stands out as one of the best.

SYMPHONY NO. 94 IN G (SURPRISE)
JOSEPH HAYDN
Largely credited with standardizing the symphony as we know it today, Haydn was a prolific composer. Of his 104

symphonies, no. 94 perhaps best highlights the humor and fun he injected into his work. Find the Sir Colin Davis–conducted, Royal Concertgebouw Orchestra–performed version (1994) and turn up the volume for the full "surprise" experience.

TRUMPET CONCERTO IN E FLAT

JOSEPH HAYDN

As a former trumpet player, perhaps my single favorite moment in classical music is the triumphant trumpet solo entrance in the first movement. While most trumpet faithful will no doubt argue that the definitive recording belongs to Maurice Andre or Wynton Marsalis, my favorite belongs to relative newcomer Tine Thing Helseth backed by the Norwegian Chamber Orchestra, recorded in 2007.

ROMANTIC PERIOD (1800–1900)

During the Romantic era, composers began to use music to fully express their emotions. While Baroque music was written to praise God and Classical music to entertain the wealthy, Romantic music was created to lament a heartbreak and subsequent drug-fueled descent into despair (as in Berlioz's *Symphonie Fantastique*) or to express elation at nature's beauty during a summer walk in the woods (as in Beethoven's Symphony no. 6, *Pastoral*). Romantic music is passionate, dramatic, and exciting—kind of like that crazy redhead you dated in college.

SYMPHONY NO. 5

LUDWIG VAN BEETHOVEN

Beethoven's Fifth is a powerful expression of his mighty yet ultimately victorious struggle with destiny. The Fifth Symphony was sometimes circulated under the name "The Symphony of Destiny" and Beethoven once explained its instantly recognizable "da da da daaa" motif in this way: *So pocht das Schicksal an die Pforte* ("Thus Destiny knocks at the door"). Experience the foreboding then triumphant musical journey with the quintessential Carlos Kleiber and Vienna Philharmonic Orchestra recording.

PIANO CONCERTO NO. I

Pyotr Ilyich Tchaikovsky

In 1958, at the height of the Cold War, a twenty-four-year-old Texan named Van Cliburn boldly traveled to Moscow. He returned a hero as Grand Prize winner of the First International Tchaikovsky Competition. A few months later he recreated his mesmerizing performance of Piano Concerto no. 1 at Carnegie Hall, recording it for posterity. Dripping with passion and fire, the Cliburn recording is one of the greatest piano concertos of all time played by a true master.

SYMPHONY NO. 9 IN E MINOR, OP. 95
(*FROM THE NEW WORLD*)

Antonín Dvořák

Dvořák's journey from his beloved Bohemia to the exciting unknown of America is mirrored in this symphony, written during his time in New York. The *New World* Symphony is equally influenced by Native American and African-American themes and nostalgia for Dvořák's Czech homeland. Enchanting, grand, idealistic, and free-spirited, *From the New World* seemingly bottles the essence of the American spirit. Fritz Reiner's recording with the Chicago Symphony Orchestra is fantastic.

Keys to a Good Listening Experience

- TAKE YOUR TIME Classical music isn't good at providing instant gratification. Make sure you have enough time to absorb the full musical piece without feeling anxious or rushed.

- EQUIPMENT MATTERS For best results, listen using high-end headphones or a premium sound system that can properly deliver the full richness, texture, and depth of the recording.

- EXERCISE YOUR MIND'S EYE Closing your eyes will heighten your aural sense and open your third eye (your mind's eye). Try to visualize the music in terms of a story or scene.

- PLAY THE SHRINK As you listen, spend time identifying specific emotions you hear in the music. Your diagnosis of the composer's state of mind will help you better understand the work.

ROMEO AND JULIET, OVERTURE-FANTASY
PYOTR ILYICH TCHAIKOVSKY

Like many other romantic era composers, Tchaikovsky was strongly influenced by Shakespeare. While Tchaikovsky also wrote works based on *The Tempest* and *Hamlet,* his musical portrayal of Verona's young, star-crossed lovers is the best known and well-loved of his Shakespearean inspired works. As you listen to the New York Philharmonic Orchestra's 2004 recording, conducted by Leonard Bernstein, try to pick up the distinct instrumental motifs of Friar Laurence, the warring families, and the lovers themselves.

QUESTION TO CONTEMPLATE In an ADD world where immediate yet often unfulfilling gratification is increasingly the norm, how might you slow down to connect with the values and emotions that make you human? Do you want to be intentional about seeking out slower, richer, fuller experiences?

GENTLEMANLY QUOTE TO REMEMBER
"Music washes away from the soul the dust of everyday life."

— G.M. Weilacher

ACTION STEP Carve out some time and explore the list of recommendations, or seek out other works that you find intriguing. After a few listens, your musical taste will begin to form. Note what resonates with you and what doesn't. If a composer, era, or instrument speaks strongly to you, dig deeper! Welcome to a lifelong journey of musical discovery.

Dine Like Royalty: Etiquette at the Dinner Table

I WAS RAISED in a home where dinner was a formal, sit-down, family affair every night. Proper table manners were taught early and reinforced regularly. Then I went to college. Free from the conventions of the family dining table and its civilized eating habits, speed and convenience quickly vaulted over grace and manners as my culinary priorities. In one season of pure laziness, I went months without eating anything that required dishes, just to avoid any cleaning. Eating became something to cram as quickly as possible into a schedule packed with classes, lacrosse practice, gym workouts, video games, and social functions. The poor habits I developed away at school were so ingrained that breaking them has been a long, arduous, and ongoing process.

After graduation I found myself in New York City, suddenly thrust into a world of client dinners, networking events, and a dating pool that demanded class and grace, while I was akin to a Neanderthal emerging from a time machine. Here are some of the lessons and tips I (re)learned the hard way.

PUMP THE BRAKES

Eat slowly. No one wants to share a table with an open-mouthed shoveler. Take a manageable bite and finish it before adding another. Chew with your mouth closed and leave room for conversation between swallows. After all, that's presumably why you've been invited for dinner.

NAPKIN NORMS

Your napkin should be folded on your lap shortly after you sit down. Use your napkin regularly throughout the meal, even if you don't think you need to. Wipe your mouth before taking a drink to avoid leaving food residue on your glass. Should you encounter a piece of bone or gristle, discreetly deposit it into your napkin and subtly request a replacement napkin from your waiter. When excusing yourself from the table, a napkin should be folded clean side up and placed to the left of your plate.

"B" FOR BREAD, "D" FOR DRINK

The sheer number of plates, glasses, and cutlery at a formal dinner can be enough to intimidate even the most confident diner. One easy trick to ensure you don't sip your neighbor's water or steal his bread is to make an OK sign with each hand. The "b" formed by your left hand tells you that your bread plate is on your left while the "d" from your right hand points the way to your drink glasses.

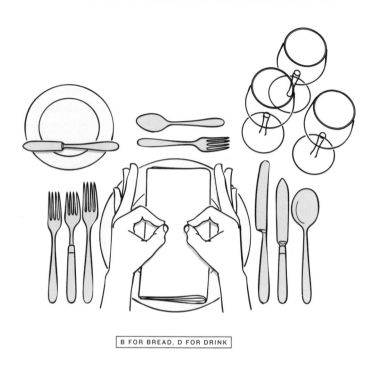

B FOR BREAD, D FOR DRINK

Silverware is arranged to be used from the outside in. Forks are placed to the left side of your plate with knives and spoons to the right (the exception is an oyster fork, which is placed on the right). Dessert spoons and forks should not be part of the table setting, but more appropriately delivered with dessert.

SILVERWARE SIGNALS

A knife and fork placed apart and pointing toward the top of the plate in a triangle indicate that you're still eating. When you're finished, signal that your plate is ready to be cleared by placing your knife and fork diagonally together on your plate approximately where the number four is on a clock face.

BREAKING BREAD

Think of your bread plate as a staging area. Use your knife to place butter onto your plate and then butter your bread from there, not from the communal butter dish. Bread should be torn by hand into smaller pieces that are then buttered individually as needed. Never butter a full slice and bite directly from it.

CUTLERY COMPETENCE

Both the American style (in which the fork is held in the left hand for cutting and switched to the right for eating) and Continental style (in which the fork is kept in the left hand for both cutting and eating) are completely acceptable. However, don't cut food into more than three pieces at a time—you are not a toddler in danger of choking. Spoon soup away from you, and if you need to tilt the bowl, angle it away from you. Used silverware should never touch the table, even when resting half on a plate or bowl.

ELBOW RULES

Keep your elbows off the table while eating. However, it is okay to place your elbows on the table during conversation between courses, or with coffee. In fact, this can often signal interest and engagement in your conversation. One place your elbows should never go is into the guests seated beside you. Tuck your elbows in and keep your movements small when cutting and eating.

SALT AND PEPPER

At the dinner table, salt and pepper are married and should always travel together. Ask for both and pass both, even if someone requests just one or the other. Don't season your food without tasting it first—this shows respect for the chef, and saves you from potentially ruining an already perfectly seasoned meal.

BE CONSISTENT

While you may just be eating dinner alone at home, be conscious of your manners nonetheless. Habits are hard to break, and manners can't be reliably switched on and off depending on your setting.

WHY TABLE MANNERS STILL MATTER

Perhaps the reason my childhood lessons in table manners didn't stick is that the only explanation I was given for their importance was "It's polite and the proper thing to do." If you require slightly more incentive to motivate your dining etiquette, here are some very practical implications:

BUSINESS BOOST OR BUST. In business, your appearance and actions are an outward representation of your work and the organization you work for. Employers get behind employees whom they can rely on as the face of the company, and are less supportive of those that can't be trusted. Clients want to be reassured that their business is in the right hands. Poor table manners can unnecessarily call into question your work ethic or aptitude. After all, if you're sloppy at the dinner table, perhaps you're also sloppy with other professional courtesies, or at the spreadsheet.

CONVERSATION KILLER. No matter how interesting your conversation might be, if food is flying in and out of your mouth, no one's really listening to you.

RESPECT. A primary goal of the gentleman is to make others feel comfortable. Through common courtesy, including table manners, we recognize the humanity in others. If we want others to treat us with respect we must first treat them with respect.

GOOD TABLE MANNERS ARE THE POLITE AND PROPER THING TO DO. As always, Mom was right.

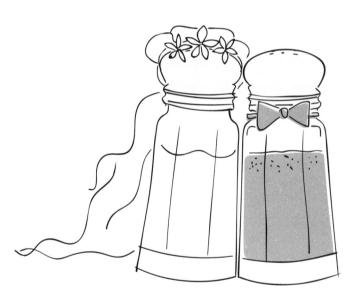

ALWAYS TOGETHER

19   DINE LIKE ROYALTY: ETIQUETTE AT THE DINNER TABLE

 QUESTION TO CONTEMPLATE What role do common courtesies, including table manners, play in a civilized society? What would a world devoid of social etiquette look like?

 GENTLEMANLY QUOTE TO REMEMBER "A man's manners are a mirror in which he shows his portrait."

— Johann Wolfgang von Goethe

 ACTION STEP It can be a helpful and eye-opening exercise to see what others see when you eat. Set up a mirror at dinner one night and watch yourself. Better yet, record video of the meal and watch it later. Then erase it quickly before it mysteriously ends up on the Internet. If you have someone in your life that you feel completely comfortable with, ask them to honestly evaluate your table manners. Just don't get offended or upset when they say you remind them of Cookie Monster.

The Confident Conversationalist

THE FRENCH are generally considered to be among the world's best conversationalists. In Paris's famed eighteenth-century salons, artists and nobles gathered for the primary purpose of open-ended discussion, a tradition that is alive and well in French institutions and cultural values to this day. In French schools, debate is compulsory, and high school graduation requires passing a written philosophy exam posing questions such as "Is it absurd to desire the impossible?" and "Are there questions that no science answers?" On warm nights it's not uncommon to find Parisians gathered on the banks of the Seine for hours of wine-fueled conversation. Simply put, the French are good at conversation because they value conversation.

A gentleman finds great value in conversation. No gentleman is an island unto himself and conversation is his passport into an eye-opening world of inspiring new ideas and knowledge. Conversation is also an opportunity for the sharing and testing of a gentleman's own ideas and knowledge, often revealing as much about himself as his partner. Conversation facilitates deeper relationships, multiplies individual potential through cocreation, and creates understanding, which is essential for change. Once a gentleman recognizes the value of conversation, becoming "good" at it requires just a little intention and practice.

FILL YOUR CONVERSATIONAL QUIVER

Conversations often begin with someone asking, in some form, "What's going on?" Consider how many times you have replied, "Nothing much. You?" This reflexive response is not only a conversation nonstarter, it's selling you short. Here are three ready trains of thought to hop on and start a fruitful conversation.

TELL A STORY

Stories are the backbone of good conversation, and personal stories humanize conversation and provide emotional touch points that allow us to connect with one another. Stories don't need to be epic to be conversation-worthy, so don't worry if you haven't climbed Kilimanjaro or performed a citizen's arrest this week. The key to good storytelling is not necessarily even content, but delivery, and good delivery requires practice. Train yourself to view day-to-day life experiences as stories, incidental or consequential. Mentally translating an experience into a story as it happens will ingrain it in your memory for later conversation. Reciting a story to yourself a few times before you tell it can help keep it concise and ensure it has a strong hook and satisfying payoff. Consider what makes the story interesting to you and you'll discover the transition from one-way storytelling to two-way conversation.

DISCUSS THE WORLD AT LARGE

Current affairs are conversational currency. Be it news, sports, entertainment, politics, or culture, these shared subjects are easily accessible conversation fodder. Your personal interests will guide what you're most inclined to talk about, but here are some additional ways to spark your knowledge and curiosity, leaving you eager for discussion.

- Download podcasts to replace music for your daily commute. Public radio can also be a great source for understanding the latest issues or unearthing interesting stories on your morning drive.

- Set up an RSS feed of content for quick digestion at lunch. Be wary of oversubscribing; the vastness of the web can quickly overwhelm your feed.

- Read. Nonfiction and fiction. Magazines and newspapers. In print and onscreen. At home or on a mobile device.

- Watch *some* TV. People love talking about their favorite shows and contrary to what Mom said, a couple hours a week won't turn your brain to mush (unless you're watching trashy reality shows). With DVR, on-demand, and mobile technology, you can now watch more efficiently and on your own schedule.

- Subscribe to print editions. The newspaper on my doorstep or magazine in my mailbox is a tangible and immediate reminder to stay informed. The act of reading information arranged on pages, especially in a newspaper, can lead you to skim or even pore over articles that you may not necessarily have clicked on as a digital link. And call me old-fashioned, but I still prefer the tactile feel of turning a page to clicking a mouse or swiping a screen.

- If you can resist the urge to go down the rabbit hole, social networks can be a great source for friend-referred articles and stories.

- Have more conversations. Discussing the contents of previous conversations is a great way to add perspective, and if it was interesting once, it stands to reason it will be again!

BE AN IDEA MAN

It's been said that small minds talk about people, moderate minds talk about events, and great minds talk about ideas. While any conversation might start off with small talk, as the conversation develops don't be shy about carrying it into the realm of issues and ideas. If your conversational partner would rather keep it light, and especially if you're headed into areas that might be controversial, don't push it, but you may also be surprised how interested they may be in an exchange of some depth. Spend time reflecting on ideas and you'll be equipped for conversations of substance, no matter what the topic.

THE WELCOME INQUISITOR

Most people prefer to talk about themselves, so being a good conversationalist is often as easy as asking the right questions and getting out of the way. One key to asking good questions is avoiding "poll" questions, in which the answer is a simple yes or no. A good example of a poll question is "Do you like *band XYZ?*" Instead, you might ask why someone likes a particular band, about his or her interpretation of a song's lyrics, or about significant memories tied to the band's music. Ask open-ended questions that are likely to elicit an emotional response and you're much more likely to kick off deeper, higher-energy, more enjoyable conversations.

LISTEN UP!

Our natural, self-centered tendency to talk instead of listen can be a stumbling block for lively and engaged conversation. While we politely nod and smile, our minds are going overtime thinking about what to say next and we inevitably miss a lot (a dismal 50 to 75 percent of the average conversation, according to studies).

Fortunately, active listening is a skill that any gentleman can practice and improve. In your next conversation, try these exercises:

- Consciously repeat the words you hear in your head to stay focused and reinforce their message.

- Make reflecting statements and ask clarifying questions: "It sounds like . . ." or "What do you mean by . . ."

- Minimize environmental distractions. Position yourself so that there aren't any visual distractions behind the speaker such as other people, TV screens, or clocks.

QUESTION TO CONTEMPLATE In any social situation there are people to avoid (the dullards, the blowhards, the steamrollers) and then there are brilliant conversationalists who enliven any conversation and are always excellent company. What can you do to improve your conversational skills and become a welcome sight at any party or gathering?

 GENTLEMANLY QUOTE TO REMEMBER "Perhaps the best conversationalist in the world is the man who helps others to talk."

— JOHN STEINBECK, *EAST OF EDEN*

 ACTION STEP View your day-to-day life as eventful, with stories to share for their own sake or as jumping-off points to other areas of interest. Help fill your conversational quiver by expanding your knowledge of current affairs. Meanwhile, work on your questioning and listening skills by attempting a conversation that is completely about the other person. Try not to talk about yourself at all. It's harder than it sounds!

21

A Gentleman Throws a Party

WHETHER FOR DINNER, drinks, or dancing, a gentleman-hosted party should reflect the character of its host— thoughtful, welcoming, and sophisticated. Facilitating a night of drunken debauchery that fuels gossip is never the goal of the gentleman host. The aim is to provide a comfortable environment for spirited, meaningful conversation, deepened friendships, and new introductions.

For the Victorian-era gentleman, throwing a fantastic party was as easy as calling on the family retainer with a request of "dinner for eight, please, Alfred." Those days are long past and the reality is that today a good party's success lies primarily on the broad shoulders of its gentlemanly host. The hard truth is that pulling off a successful event requires a lot of care, intention, and thought. The result, however, is absolutely worth the effort, and with a few strategies and advance planning, the modern gentleman can pull off a memorable and meaningful gathering without feeling in over his head.

T MINUS TWO WEEKS - GUEST LIST AND INVITATIONS

Think about whom you'd like to invite. The size of the party is an important consideration when populating the guest list. A smaller, more intimate party requires a more thoughtful pairing of personalities. Balance common interests with stimulating differences. The goal is for your guests to complement one another rather than compete with one another. At a larger party, while the initial guest list requires less finesse it may require more attention to on-the-spot matchmaking and introductions.

Once the guest list has been finalized, it's time to spread the word. In today's digital age, more often than not invitations are sent via email, a digital invite service such as Evite, or (gasp!) even text message. However, the modern gentleman can set himself apart and let his guests know how valued they are by extending invitations the "right" way—with a phone call or written note. Invitations should go out about two weeks in advance of the event when possible. Any less than a week in advance and you risk implying that your guests aren't valued or that they might be a last-minute replacement.

Keep your guests from potentially uncomfortable situations by making your invitations as clear and specific as possible. In addition to time and place, include the type of party, particularly specifying if food will be served. Add a contact number, a prompt for reply (if required), and any pertinent travel or parking information. Depending on your crowd and the nature of the event, you also might want to indicate the appropriate attire.

T MINUS ONE WEEK - MENU PLANNING

For a cocktail party, prepare for differing tastes by presenting

Dinner Party Tips

- If the microwave is generally the most used appliance in your kitchen, you're probably ill-equipped to cook for a large party. If you find yourself in need of oversized pots and pans, extra serving platters, or specialty cooking tools, consider renting them from a local catering supply company. If you really don't cook, consider having the food catered as well.

- At a dinner party, make sure your menu provides a generous contrast of flavors, colors, and textures. Your guests' taste buds are destined for flavor fatigue by a menu of tomato soup, followed by a salad topped by bright tomatoes and spaghetti with tomato sauce. If you're serving duck à l'orange, you might want to reconsider pre-dinner blood orange margaritas. In the same way, contrast the crisp crunch of a fried appetizer with a baked main course. Play with crisp vs. soft, chewy vs. creamy, thick vs. thin, and keep your guests anticipating and guessing.

- Despite all your diligent planning, if the first knock on the door is approaching too quickly, stop working to shower and dress. It's acceptable, if not ideal, to finish preparations once guests arrive. It's not okay to shower.

- Need a sous chef in the kitchen? Want to offer valet parking? Dreading the solo post-party cleanup? Extra help isn't necessarily a budget buster. Many college students might be willing to help out for $10–$20 an hour.

- If a guest brings a gift, there is no need for you to write a thank-you note as that would amount to thanking him for thanking you.

a range of alcohol types and appropriate mixers, and consider offering a specialty cocktail or two (see Chapter 11). Don't neglect to include options for any nondrinkers in attendance. It's always nice to serve a few snacks or hors d'oeuvres, and the guest arriving with an empty stomach will thank you.

If you're serving dinner, save your guests from possible embarrassment by inquiring about food preferences, allergies, or restrictions in advance. Carefully think through your menu and take into account the capacities of your kitchen. Underestimating refrigerator space, cookware requirements, oven timing, and/or serving needs can sink a promising party at the moment of truth. If you're not an experienced cook, now is probably not the time to get ambitious. Just keep things simple and go with what you know. Make a list of everything you'll need, grouped by shopping location (grocery store, home goods store, liquor store, etc).

T MINUS TWO OR THREE DAYS - SHOPPING

Unless your menu calls for ingredients that must be as fresh as possible (seafood comes to mind) get your shopping done early and leave the day of the party free for last-second inevitabilities. In addition to the ingredients from your menu, remember to stock up on household goods like toilet paper and paper towels, as well as coffee for any lingering late-night revelers.

T MINUS ONE DAY - CLEANING AND PREPPING

Your home will tell your guests a lot about you — don't let "messy" make the list. As men, we often confuse "tidy" with "clean," but now is not the time to make that mistake. You'll want to dust, vacuum, and scrub in addition to your usual stacking and shuffling. Pay special attention to the bathrooms.

The privacy of a locked door may give inquisitive guests the temptation to poke around.

Also use the day before for any food prep that can safely be done ahead of time. Many desserts and appetizers are fine made beforehand and refrigerated. Double-check your dishes, silverware, glasses, and napkins by setting the table ahead of time. Finally, make sure you have enough ice made and start chilling beer and white wine.

T MINUS FOUR HOURS - PREGAME ORGANIZATION

Trim meat, stuff birds, apply marinades or rubs; wash, peel, and chop vegetables; and organize a *mise en place* — a culinary term to describe arranging all the ingredients you'll need to cook quickly and efficiently. Line up all the ingredients you'll need for each step, returning perishables to the fridge but leaving the appropriate tools in place. A little pregame measuring and organization will save precious time once the pots and pans start flying for real.

T MINUS ONE HOUR - FINAL DETAILS

The moment of truth is approaching, but your prior planning means there isn't much left to do. Take care of any last-minute details: slice lemons and limes, chill glasses, fill the ice bucket, put on some music, light candles, open the wine to "breathe," and get dressed (maybe you should get dressed first).

DING-DONG - TIME TO BE A HEROIC HOST

Try to greet each guest and have a drink in their hand within five minutes of their arrival. This can be a challenge at larger parties. Enlist the help of a significant other or close friend to man the door while you greet, fix drinks, and make introductions.

In a small gathering, lead each new arrival into the party and introduce him to everyone personally. At larger parties, greet the guest and then introduce him to a small group already engaged in conversation or pass him along to someone he knows who can handle further introductions. Your goal with each introduction is to provide a smooth transition into conversation. Therefore each introduction should include relevant information about each party as a catalyst for conversation.

> *"John Smith, this is Thomas Chang. Thomas is an assistant DA here in New York. He's also an outdoor survival expert and recently summited Everest. Thomas, John is an old college friend and lacrosse teammate. He just moved here with his wife to join the New York Philharmonic Orchestra as its new principal oboe."*

Remember that as host, your primary concern is the well-being of your guests, not your own enjoyment. Don't get too engrossed in any single conversation, at least early in the night. Spread your attention broadly so that everyone feels valued and welcome. Keep a constant eye open for signs of boredom or isolation. If you spot someone by themselves, invite them into conversation with another guest or enlist their help with passing food. Likewise, be on the lookout for conversations past their expiration date. At some point in the evening you may need to rescue a helpless guest from an overly aggressive salesman or tactfully intervene in a heated political discussion. You are responsible for the experiences, both good and bad, of every guest under your roof.

Lastly, have fun, but stay sober. Nothing will damage your ability to be a gracious and attentive host as much as too much alcohol.

A GENTLEMAN THROWS A PARTY

QUESTION TO CONTEMPLATE If you believe that personal relationships are a priority in your life, what are you doing to intentionally deepen friendships, facilitate new connections, and encourage camaraderie? If you truly want more meaningful relationships, isn't it incumbent on you to make it happen?

GENTLEMANLY QUOTE TO REMEMBER "If more of us valued food and cheer and song above hoarded gold, it would be a merrier world."

— J.R.R. Tolkien

ACTION STEP Tired of once-vibrant friendships now characterized by passing small talk or the occasional email? Want to develop real connections with new acquaintances, colleagues, or classmates? Take ownership of developing and maintaining your personal relationships by hosting a great party!

A Morning Routine for Daily Domination

EVERYONE LOVES THE SNOOZE BUTTON, but push it one too many times and you'll find yourself in a frantic scramble to get out the door on time. A stressful morning without routine can leave you feeling unsettled and unprepared, like you're playing catch-up for the rest of the day. However, a good morning routine will ground you and set the tone for daily productivity and vitality. As a modern gentleman there's a lot on your plate, so make sure you're set up to dominate life with an efficient and effective morning routine.

PREEMPTIVE PLANNING

A good morning routine actually starts before you head to bed. Deciding what to wear in the morning can add undue stress and eat up valuable time. Choosing your outfit and doing any ironing or steaming the night before will result in one

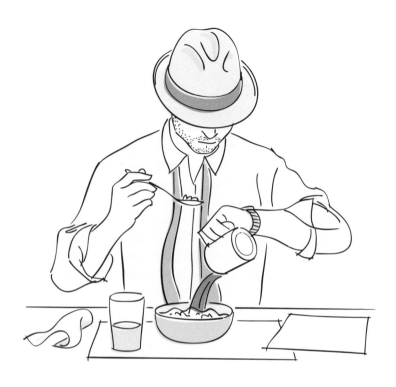

MORNING RUSH HOUR

less decision for your groggy, pre-coffee condition. Save your closet from manic morning messiness and ensure you leave put-together and wrinkle-free with some presleep prep work.

NO BEEPS DURING DEEP SLEEP

Sometimes you wake up after nine hours of sleep feeling absolutely exhausted. Other mornings you spring out of bed after six hours of sleep feeling completely refreshed. The distinction is most likely not in *how* you slept, but *when* you were woken. During sleep we cycle through five stages, with a complete cycle taking about 90 to 110 minutes. Stages one and two are considered "light" sleep, stages three and four are considered "deep" sleep, and stage five is REM (rapid eye movement), the stage in which we dream. Nature intended for us to wake during "light" sleep, and when we do we feel rested, alert, and ready to hit the ground running. Conversely, if we are unnaturally jarred out of "deep" sleep, we feel groggy, lethargic, and ready to hit nothing but the snooze button.

There are a few methods that can help time your morning rise to coincide with sleep stages one or two. The most effective, but expensive, option is to purchase a gadget that tracks your sleep cycles and wakes you only during optimal "light" sleep. Wristwatch-like motion monitors and head-bands that monitor brain activity have proven effective for people without severe sleep problems (insomnia, apnea, etc.), but are somewhat involved. A cheaper option is to estimate your sleep patterns based on ninety-minute cycles. Resources like www.sleepyti.me provide "best guess" wake-up times based on the time you go to bed or best bed times based on what time you want to wake up. You can also try setting two alarms: your normal alarm and a very light alarm, set to go off thirty minutes earlier. The theory is that the light alarm will only wake you during "light" sleep, while your normal alarm acts as a backup.

JUMP-START YOUR INTERNAL SYSTEM

After sleeping, the body's tissues are in dire need of hydration and cleansing. Warm lemon water is the ideal way to hydrate and oxygenate, kick-starting clean cellular energy production and flushing accumulated toxins. Morning lemon water also helps activate your digestive system, readying it for the day's meals, and gives your system a nice boost of vitamin C.

To make lemon water, simply heat water in a kettle or microwave until hot, but not scalding, just short of boiling. Squeeze half a lemon into the hot water and add a squeeze of honey. Stir and enjoy. Always use fresh lemons for full vitamin, enzyme, and antioxidant power. Wait about fifteen to thirty minutes for your system to fully wake up and reboot before eating your normal, healthy breakfast.

WAKE UP YOUR CORE

Before you get in the shower, do a few quick sets of push-ups to get your blood pumping. Reenergizing the core muscles in your chest, back, and abdominals will improve your posture—boosting your height and confidence—for the rest of the day. And if you don't make it to the gym later, you can rest easy knowing you've already gotten a little bit of PT.

HEAD TO TOE

If you find yourself constantly pressed for time in the morning, don't stumble directly from your bed to the shower. In your half-asleep state you can waste a lot of time and water standing comatose under the hot spray. When you do get in, shower with purpose. Develop a process and think of each step as a task to be completed. I find that starting from the top of my head and working my way down helps me stay focused and not forget anything. Shampoo, conditioner, face wash, body wash, rinse, and I can be in and out in five minutes. If you really love hanging out under the hot water, and who can blame you, multitask by adding teeth brushing and/or shaving to your in-shower routine.

FEED THE BEAST

You've heard it once; you've heard it a hundred times. Breakfast is the most important meal of the day. Focus on healthy, slow-burn foods like whole grains, lean protein, and fresh fruits and vegetables. A vegetable omelet or a bowl of steel-cut oats with fruit and low-fat yogurt are great ways to break your overnight fast. If you've recently joined the juicing craze or can't stomach solid food early in the morning, opt for a fresh-squeezed veggie and fruit juice or quickly blended smoothie. Eating a healthy breakfast is linked to higher levels of concentration, productivity, and even weight loss. If you don't think you have time for breakfast, make time.

PREPARE YOUR MIND

Before you step across the threshold and into the fray of hectic, modern life, take just a few moments to center your mind. Think about the day's schedule and the important things you want to accomplish. Close your eyes and take a few deep breaths in quiet solitude. Maybe browse the newspaper, or spend some time journaling. Talk with your kids or chat with your spouse. Remind yourself of all the things for which you're thankful. And then walk out the door, refreshed, energized, and motivated to conquer your world.

QUESTION TO CONTEMPLATE How is your time spent between waking up and walking out the front door? Are you setting yourself up for a successful day or starting behind the eight ball?

 GENTLEMANLY QUOTE TO REMEMBER "Morning is when the wick is lit. A flame ignited, the day delighted with heat and light, we start the fight for something more than before."

— JEB DICKERSON

 ACTION STEP Integrate some or all of the suggestions in this chapter into your morning routine. The development of good morning habits often falls into the category of "great in theory, hard in practice." Discipline yourself for a week of earlier rising and more structured mornings. See if you notice any changes in your mind-set, productivity, or vitality. It might be hard to believe, but your body will adjust. What might require tremendous will power today will become effortless routine tomorrow.

Poetry for Men

BY ALL ACCOUNTS, Theodore Roosevelt was a man's man: a big-game hunter, avid explorer, and rough-riding soldier. Yet amid his testosterone-driven exploits and adventures, one of his fondest passions was poetry. In fact, during his tenure as president, Roosevelt instituted government positions exclusively for writing new poetry, and recited a few verses and rhymes to his children each night before bed. And he himself had the poetic gift: his speech "The Man in the Arena" remains one of the most well-known and masculine pieces of poetry to this day.

Poetry once occupied a position at the apex of cultural masculinity. That it has since become perceived as unmanly defies logic, fact, and common sense. After all, poetry can trace its roots to the tales of warrior heroes such as Achilles

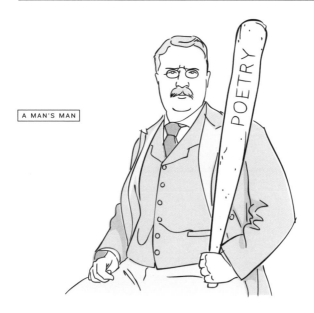

and Beowulf, and it explores the most influential aspects of life, from love and war to purpose and destiny, adventure and friendship to mortality and legacy. What could be more masculine?

Here are a few verses that will restore your manly faith in the art of poetry:

IF . . .

BY RUDYARD KIPLING

Few words have ever captured the essence of manhood quite so wholly and eloquently. Like the ultimate father-son talk, Kipling's words are full of passion, inspiration, and wisdom that can be applied to almost any circumstance a man might face.

If you want to live life to the fullest . . . if you want to be a better version of yourself . . . if you want to be a gentleman . . . then "If . . ."

≈ ≈ ≈ ≈

If you can keep your head when all about you
Are losing theirs and blaming it on you,
If you can trust yourself when all men doubt you,
But make allowance for their doubting too;

If you can wait and not be tired by waiting,
Or being lied about, don't deal in lies,
Or being hated, don't give way to hating,
And yet don't look too good, nor talk too wise:

If you can dream — and not make dreams your master;
If you can think — and not make thoughts your aim;
If you can meet with Triumph and Disaster
And treat those two impostors just the same;

If you can bear to hear the truth you've spoken
Twisted by knaves to make a trap for fools,
Or watch the things you gave your life to broken,
And stoop and build 'em up with worn-out tools:

If you can make one heap of all your winnings
And risk it on one turn of pitch-and-toss,
And lose, and start again at your beginnings
And never breathe a word about your loss;

If you can force your heart and nerve and sinew
To serve your turn long after they are gone,
And so hold on when there is nothing in you
Except the Will which says to them: 'Hold on!'

If you can talk with crowds and keep your virtue,
Or walk with kings — nor lose the common touch,
If neither foes nor loving friends can hurt you,
If all men count with you, but none too much;

If you can fill the unforgiving minute
With sixty seconds' worth of distance run —
Yours is the Earth and everything that's in it,
And — which is more — you'll be a Man, my son!

≈ ≈ ≈ ≈

INVICTUS

BY WILLIAM ERNEST HENLEY

Adversity is a harsh reality of life, indiscriminate in its reach
and merciless in its effect. Rich or poor, young or old, rising
star or fading supernova, adversity will assuredly strike every
man at some point in life. One clear mark of a gentleman is his
response to life's body blows. "Invictus" presents a picture of
character, perseverance, and sheer will that every man should
aspire to when faced with "the fell clutch of circumstance,"
"the bludgeonings of chance," and "the menace of the years."

≈ ≈ ≈ ≈

Out of the night that covers me,
Black as the pit from pole to pole,
I thank whatever gods may be
For my unconquerable soul.

In the fell clutch of circumstance
I have not winced nor cried aloud.
Under the bludgeonings of chance
My head is bloody, but unbowed.

Beyond this place of wrath and tears
Looms but the Horror of the shade,
And yet the menace of the years
Finds, and shall find, me unafraid.

It matters not how strait the gate,
How charged with punishments the scroll.
I am the master of my fate:
I am the captain of my soul.

LIVE YOUR LIFE
BY CHIEF TECUMSEH

Legacy. Every gentleman wants to leave one. To know that
our lives mattered and that we left a mark upon the world for
the better, even if in just some small way. To be remembered
fondly and missed deeply. Regret. We all want to avoid it. To
live our lives in the same way as we would if given a mulli-
gan at mortality. To take advantage of all of life's opportunities and rise up to face all of its challenges. Chief Tecumseh
lays out the road map for a life well-lived: pride tempered by
humility, equal respect for oneself and others, gratitude for
life regardless of circumstance, the pursuit of purpose over
fear, and a heart for service over self. Follow the chief's advice
and your life will surely be marked by legacy, not regret.

So live your life that the fear of death can never enter
    your heart.

Trouble no one about their religion; respect others in their view, and demand that they respect yours.

Love your life, perfect your life, beautify all things in your life.

Seek to make your life long and its purpose in the service of your people.

Prepare a noble death song for the day when you go over the great divide.

Always give a word or a sign of salute when meeting or passing a friend, even a stranger, when in a lonely place.

Show respect to all people and grovel to none.

When you arise in the morning give thanks for the food and for the joy of living.

If you see no reason for giving thanks, the fault lies only in yourself.

Abuse no one and no thing, for abuse turns the wise ones to fools and robs the spirit of its vision.

When it comes your time to die, be not like those whose hearts are filled with the fear of death, so that when their time comes they weep and pray for a little more time to live their lives over again in a different way.

Sing your death song and die like a hero going home.

≈ ≈ ≈ ≈

QUESTION TO CONTEMPLATE What are your perceptions of poetry? What masculine qualities can you identify, and relate to, in poetry?

GENTLEMANLY QUOTE TO REMEMBER "A poet's work is to name the unnamable, to point at frauds, to take sides, start arguments, shape the world, and stop it going to sleep."

— SALMAN RUSHDIE

ACTION STEP Find a poem that challenges or resonates with you. Write out a copy of the poem and carry it in your pocket for a week. Every time you reach into your pocket, take out the page and recite the poem to yourself until you've committed it to memory. Share it with someone who might be similarly moved by it.

Start an Honorable Gentleman's Club

BEFORE THE TERM "GENTLEMAN'S CLUB" became a promotional euphemism with less-than-gentlemanly connotations, it described a place where men bonded by a common interest or background could share information, ideas, experiences, and otherwise socialize in comfort and privacy. The late nineteenth century is considered the height of club influence, but traditional gentleman's clubs are once again gaining popularity.

While the most prominent clubs still maintain strict, often-secretive membership requirements and long waiting lists, the aspiring gentleman clubber doesn't need a Gilded Age surname or bursting bank account to enjoy the invigorating camaraderie that the best clubs provide. In fact, starting your own club is easy, affordable, and the best way to ensure the club's culture and membership are what you're looking for.

DEFINE YOUR RAISON D'ETRE

The first order of business is identifying the purpose of your club. The most successful clubs are created around an underlying commonality that provides an immediate bond for its members. Traditionally clubs were centered on political affiliation, industry, or military service, but your club can be focused on any shared hobby, interest, or passion. Whether specific (e.g., whiskey tasting) or broad (e.g., cocktails in general), your choice should be something you're passionate about and that is enhanced when shared with others. For example, if you crave substantive, intellectual discussion of current events and how you can impact the pertinent issues, perhaps you can start "The Current Club of YOUR HOME-TOWN," in which members take turns presenting a pressing issue and their point of view for discussion with the group at large. Beyond the "what," also consider the "why" behind your new club—your mission statement. Art may bring you together, but are you a community of artists looking for inspiration and encouragement, or art enthusiasts interested in a place to discover, discuss, and critique?

THE RULE OF THREE

King Solomon once wisely declared that a cord of three strands is not easily broken, and anyone familiar with carpentry knows that a three-legged stool is strong and stable, unlikely to tip or wobble. While not a hard and fast rule, three is also an ideal number of founding club members. A club of two doesn't quite seem official and requires perfect attendance for a meeting to happen. A foursome means no forced majority in voting and can naturally produce internal partnerships, which can create division. If you can't find at least two

Not quite ready to start a club but still looking for one to call home? Check out these interesting options:

THE CIRCUMNAVIGATORS CLUB. Founded in 1902, this international organization exists to "recognize excellence and provide a platform for the exchange of ideas among members." Membership is only open to those who have completed at least one complete circumnavigation of the globe, crossing every meridian of longitude in the same direction (not necessarily in one trip).

THE LONDON LOUNGE CLOTH CLUB. Born out of London Lounge, an online forum "dedicated to the discussion of the Bespoke Arts," the Cloth Club is a collection of gentlemen who collaboratively design and commission high-quality suiting fabric. The final designs are manufactured by some of the world's finest weavers, giving Cloth Club members access to exclusive, unique fabrics for distinctive bespoke clothing.

THE DULL MEN'S CLUB. This thoroughly tongue-in-cheek club exists as "a place for dull men to feel at home, to feel comfortable, and to share safe excitement." Founded in New York City in the mid-80s, the DMC, among other boring things, keeps track of the rotational direction of over four hundred luggage carousels in airports all over the world.

other people as fired up about your club's concept as you are, it's probably time to reconsider your vision.

A CLUB NEEDS A CLUBHOUSE

Once you've found a purpose and a few founding members,

it's time to find a place where all that purpose will go down. The possibilities are endless: a local bar, someone's garage, your office, a public park, that vacant storefront on Main Street, a hotel conference room, a moonlit wooded clearing. If geographic logistics require you might even create a virtual clubhouse online via video chat. Use your imagination and don't be scared to seek out ideal yet improbable venues—worst case scenario, you're told no, and move on.

CLUB SWAG-GER

One of the primary benefits of club membership is camaraderie among members, and assorted club gear can help facilitate a feeling of inclusion and community. Plus it's just downright cool having something exclusive. Design a club insignia or logo and have fun with it. Order custom regimental-style ties or lapel pins. Add a touch of clubman class to your correspondence with custom stationery or calling cards.

FORMAL FORESIGHT

It may seem silly, especially if you only have a few members, but establishing formal processes for your fledgling club is important. If your club takes off, figuring things out on the fly is a recipe for discord and potential dissolution. Keep a formal calendar and agenda. Establishing consistent meetings is essential for maintaining the momentum and motivation in a club's early days. Vote in officers and create a set of bylaws that state how new members will be introduced, if dues will be collected, and how money will be spent. If money is collected, consider registering your club as a legal entity and opening a club bank account. A little early planning will ensure you have a strong foundation for future growth and success.

24 START AN HONORABLE GENTLEMAN'S CLUB

QUESTION TO CONTEMPLATE What in life are you passionate about, interested in exploring further, or excited to share with others? Close your eyes and visualize a few versions of your ideal day off. What are you doing, and would sharing any of the activities with others enhance the experience?

GENTLEMANLY QUOTE TO REMEMBER "As iron sharpens iron, so one man sharpens another."

—Proverbs 27:17

ACTION STEP Become a modern clubman by joining a club or starting your own. If you need some inspiration for your club, look through the subjects covered in this book for gentlemanly topics from art appreciation to bespoke suiting.

The Sartorial Matchmaker: Pattern Combinations that Work, for Work

MANY MEN are stuck in a sartorial rut. They return day after day to tried and true (read: safe and boring) combinations like a drab uniform of monotony. Dressing conservatively or having a standard "go-to" isn't necessarily bad (one of the most stylish men I know wears a navy suit and open-collared white button-down as his calling card *every* day) but it's unfortunate when men feel they have no choice because they don't know how to successfully mix and match different patterns. If you've ever felt imprisoned by a fear of clashing, prepare to be set free.

Sure, you can always safely match a solid or two with a single pattern — a solid tie on a striped dress shirt under a solid suit or a bold gingham shirt with a solid blazer and tie, for example — but that's not why you're reading this chapter, is it? Let's move on to more worrisome yet exciting prospects, shall we? Class is now in session.

PATTERN MATCHING 101: TWO PATTERNS OF THE SAME DESIGN

The first step towards pattern enlightenment is learning how to combine two patterns of the same design, such as a striped tie with a striped dress shirt or a houndstooth tie with a plaid suit. The key to combining two patterns of the same design is keeping the relative size of the two patterns as different as possible. Without an adequate contrast in scale, two similarly sized patterns of the same design can create an unfavorable illusion of movement or vibration.

THREE WAYS TO ROCK THE LOOK:

- Pair a wide-spaced pinstripe suit with a closer Bengal stripe dress shirt and a solid tie.
- Showcase a bold, wide-spaced Repp tie against a smaller pencil stripe dress shirt.
- Match a mini-houndstooth check tie on a white dress shirt with a much larger-proportioned glen plaid suit.

PATTERN MATCHING 201: TWO DIFFERENT PATTERNS

The guideline for mixing two different patterns is the inverse of mixing two patterns of the same design. While the goal in mixing two stripes, for instance, is contrasting their scale, the

Other Sartorial Rules...and How to Break Them

While following rules will make sure you don't stand out for the wrong reason, dressing by the book will never let you stand out for the right reason. Style means knowing how to break rules correctly and every gentleman should have at least a touch of style.

RULE: Always match your sock color to your pants.
HOW TO BREAK THE RULE: Add a subtle touch of color to your look by wearing a pair of socks that pick up color from somewhere else in your outfit. Matching color from your shirt, tie, or pocket square will ensure you look put-together without being boring.

RULE: Your belt must always match your shoe color.
HOW TO BREAK THE RULE: With brown leather, your shoes and belt should be generally in the same family but don't stress about perfectly matching shades. In fact, an exact match can often look a bit forced. For a bolder look, match nontraditional colors; for example, gray shoes look great with a black or navy belt. With nontraditional colors, focus on complementing, not matching. One combination where the rule definitely does apply? Mixing black and brown.

RULE: Younger men shouldn't wear double-breasted suits.
HOW TO BREAK THE RULE: Traditionally, the extra width and bulk of double-breasted suits was thought to dominate the younger man's frame but today the flair of doubling up is accessible to all with slim, sharply tailored silhouettes.

RULE: Never wear brown in town.
HOW TO BREAK THE RULE: For most of the nineteenth and twentieth centuries, men would only wear brown suits while in the country or on a farm. Who still wears a suit on a farm? Wear brown proudly, in town or out.

goal in mixing two different patterns is to keep them close in size.

The exception to the rule is when dealing with small patterns. For example, a very narrowly spaced striped shirt combined with a small foulard print tie creates the same optical discord we seek to avoid with two similarly proportioned patterns of the same design. Therefore, very small patterns must be offset with much larger ones whether they are of the same design or different.

THREE WAYS TO ROCK THE LOOK:

- A light windowpane shirt looks great contrasted against a bold, chunky, diagonal-striped tie.
- Combine a white shirt with a plaid suit and a tie whose stripes are equally spaced to the suit's plaid pattern.
- A pinstripe suit is well-suited for a checked dress shirt and solid-color tie.

PATTERN MATCHING 301: THREE DIFFERENT PATTERNS

High risk and high reward await the intrepid dresser who dares to wear three or more patterns together. If successful, such a man could find himself in the rarefied sartorial company of the Prince of Wales, Fred Astaire, Gianni Agnelli, and the Duke of Windsor (all of whom were fond of wearing three, four, or even five patterns at a time).

When two of the three patterns are the same design, follow the rule for matching two similar designs first, then add a third design that complements both. For example, you might pair a large check, small check, and large stripe or a large stripe, small stripe, and large paisley.

When mixing three patterns of the same design, scale again is our guide. All three patterns, although similar in

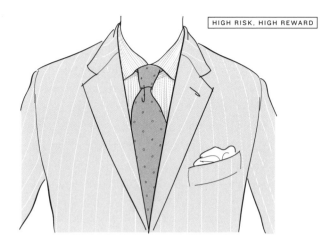

design, must be significantly different in scale to achieve appropriate balance.

THREE WAYS TO ROCK THE LOOK:

- Pair a wide-spaced pinstripe suit with a closer pencil-stripe dress shirt and a large foulard print tie.
- Graduate checks from smallest to largest starting with a small-pattern Tattersall shirt, a larger houndstooth check jacket, and a bold plaid tie.
- Wear a polka-dot tie with a Bengal stripe shirt and a flannel wool glen plaid suit for a cheeky, yet genteel look.

PATTERN MATCHING 401: FOUR OR MORE PATTERNS (INDEPENDENT STUDY)

Truly, there are no rules to guide you from this point on, only inspiration. Fred Astaire once compared dressing well to putting on a show: practice and rehearsal are necessary to achieve greatness. Spend some time in your closet "practicing" the art of dressing well. Mix and match at will, break some rules, and see what works for you. Good luck!

THE SARTORIAL MATCHMAKER: PATTERN COMBINATIONS THAT WORK, FOR WORK

QUESTION TO CONTEMPLATE Am I making full use of the value and potential already in my wardrobe? If I learn how to successfully combine patterns, how will that confidence not only expand my style but also improve the ROI of past and future clothing purchases?

GENTLEMANLY QUOTE TO REMEMBER "Be daring, be different, be impractical, be anything that will assert integrity of purpose and imaginative vision against the play-it-safers, the creatures of the commonplace, the slaves of the ordinary."

— CECIL BEATON

ACTION STEP Armed with your newfound confidence and knowledge for pattern matching, go to your closet and combine two or more elements that you've never worn together.

How to Build and Maintain a Powerful Network

WITH THE PROLIFERATION and popularity of online social networks, it's not uncommon today to find someone claiming two hundred, five hundred, or even a thousand-plus friends. But can online connections consummated with a few clicks of a mouse be considered true friendships? And despite the aid of technology that makes keeping in touch quicker and easier than ever, do humans even have the capacity to maintain hundreds of meaningful relationships?

According to Robin Dunbar, Professor of Evolutionary Anthropology at the University of Oxford, the answer to both questions is no. Dunbar has spent more than twenty years exploring social group dynamics among primates and humans. His research suggests that there is a cognitive limit on the number of stable social relationships we are able to maintain. According to Dunbar, our social capacity is biologically

How to Make Social Media Work for You

- **MAKE TWO-WAY CONVERSATION.** The majority of status updates and tweets are conversation nonstarters. Encourage virtual interaction by asking interesting questions or posting thought-provoking videos or articles. Online conversations can often roll naturally into richer offline discussions.

- **BEWARE OF RABBIT-HOLING.** It's extremely easy to waste a couple hours virtually looking in on people with whom you've long since lost touch or only met a couple times. Wouldn't it be better to invest in a real relationship by using that time for a phone call or planning a get-together?

- **LIMIT YOUR SOCIAL NETWORK FRIEND LIST TO 150.** You'll ensure that the only news and updates you'll see will be from people you genuinely care for. Likewise, you can make certain that your own posts are only seen by those with whom you have a meaningful relationship. This may seem like a drastic step, but it is one that will make your online time more efficient and relevant.

limited by neocortex size to approximately 150 relationships, a number commonly referred to as "Dunbar's number."

The significance of 150 as the optimal number for community can be traced throughout history. Hunter-gatherer societies, from Southern Africa's Bushmen to the Native Americans, naturally grouped in communities of 150. One hundred and fifty is estimated to be the size of a Neolithic farming village as well as the splitting point for Hutterite colonies and Amish settlements. The basic unit size in the Roman army and most modern militaries approximates Dunbar's number. And when Bill Gore founded Gore-Tex, he discovered that once factories exceeded 150 employees, productivity and morale quickly declined. Gore capped factory size at 150 and the resulting company culture remains a case study in employee buy-in and loyalty to this day.

The ideal of "150" has profound implications for the modern gentleman networker. We all know the importance of a network: it's how we find jobs, romantic relationships, and social interaction. However, often the effort we put forth in managing our network does not equate with the value it represents. It's time to take charge of your personal 150 and maximize the value of your network.

The first thing to understand about your 150 is that it is dynamic. Imagine slicing open an onion to reveal its many layers. Just like an onion, your network is layered with contacts arranged into radiating groups. At the center are your core relationships, the closest five or so people you know. As you move out the layers get larger and the relationships less important. As a general rule there are layers at 5, 15, 50, and 150. The constant movement within and between layers is dependent on a number of factors. Distance and time push relationships out. Nonphysical interaction (phone, email, social media) slows the rate of outward movement. Physical, face-to-face interaction draws relationships in. New introductions appear, and disregarded acquaintances drop off. You have a choice: let the constant flux happen organically or actively and strategically manage the flow.

Step one in managing your network is identifying your current 150. Compile a list by exporting your social network friend list, email address book, and cell phone contacts. Two criteria can help you cull the list. First, look for people you would feel comfortable asking a significant favor of and who in turn would feel comfortable asking a similar favor of you. Second, a strong shared history is important and can keep even the most ignored relationship on the periphery of your 150. Be honest with yourself as you go through the exercise.

Think about what you want from your network and evaluate the strength of your list against those criteria. If you are an aspiring fashion designer, are the design and fashion worlds well represented? Like to rock climb on the weekends but have a list filled with foodies? If you're on the fast track to the boardroom, you probably want to have at least a few corporate heavy hitters on board. Is a robust list of professional contacts a priority? Do you have to rub shoulders with key influencers, or do you prefer a more low-key crowd? When evaluating your connections, keep in mind the 150 of your 150. By being strategic about second-degree relationships you can really amplify the power of your network.

Whether your goal is to pull a key acquaintance from the outer layers towards the center or strengthen a closely established friendship already at the core, here are the keys to deepening relationships and getting the most out of your 150:

PHYSICAL PROXIMITY IS VITALLY IMPORTANT. Relationship growth happens most through in-person interaction. Online social networks, email, and phone calls are good for preventing relationships from decaying over time, but aren't so great for developing long-lasting bonds. No matter how many times you "Like" Tiger's status updates, if you don't get together for a round of golf sooner or later, your relationship will slowly but surely work its way through the layers of your network until it finally drops out of your 150 (the exception are family relationships, which generally seem immune to the adverse effect of distance and time).

ENDORPHINS CEMENT STRONG RELATIONAL BONDS. Endorphins are a powerful mechanism for keeping relationships together. By sharing an endorphin-rich experience with someone, you create memories that last a lifetime. Physical presence increases endorphins. Laughter is a fantastic trigger of endorphins. Exercise is another well-known endorphin liberator. New experiences, especially challenging or risky ones like adventure sports or thrill-seeking activities like skydiving, open the endorphin floodgates. Ever notice how safely emerging from a dangerous situation often results in laughter? That's the endorphins at work in your body.

FAVORS PAY OFF. Do as many favors as possible. When you go out of your way to help someone, a sense of obligation (born out of fondness, not guilt) is ingrained in the relationship and strengthens the bond. Plus, building up a store of goodwill is a good idea; you never know when it will be your turn to need a favor.

WELCOME DIVERSITY INTO YOUR 150. If your 150 all share similar interests, work in the same fields, and live in the same places, you won't have strong bridges into different worlds. When it comes to finding new jobs, ideas, insights, or knowledge, a homogeneous network isn't a very helpful one.

HOW TO BUILD AND MAINTAIN A POWERFUL NETWORK

QUESTION TO CONTEMPLATE What do you want from your network? Does your 150 deliver? How can it be improved?

GENTLEMANLY QUOTE TO REMEMBER "He who hath many friends, hath none."

— ARISTOTLE

ACTION STEP Pick one or more relationships that you want to move toward or keep near the center of your 150. Plan something that will deepen the relationship(s). Get together for a whiskey tasting, spend a weekend learning how to ice climb, go to a comedy club, take in a jazz show, or do the person(s) a significant favor.

Whisk(e)y: The Water of Life

SMOKE, MOSS, HONEY, AND FRUIT. Vanilla, pineapple, cocoa, and nutmeg. Seaweed, tobacco, leather, and grass. Hay, raisins, licorice, and . . . nail polish remover? Yes, these are just a small sampling of the descriptions found scattered throughout the tasting notes of makers and tasters of the world's most complex alcohol, whiskey. That such varied complexity of flavors and aromas can be created from just four ingredients (grain, yeast, water, and time) is a remarkable testament to the ingenuity of man.

Originally developed in the Middle Ages for medicinal purposes, whiskey's earliest name was *uisge beatha*, Gaelic for "water of life." By the time King Henry VIII dissolved the monasteries, sending the monks and their distillery knowledge out into the secular world, whiskey was already being enjoyed by the healthy and sick alike. Whiskey was used as currency in Revolutionary America, and following his presidency George Washington even operated his own distillery (newly reopened in 2006). Over the years, whiskey has survived taxation, revolution, and even prohibition. Today, interest in whiskey, and single-malt Scotch whisky in particular, has never been higher, and no other drink is more closely associated with the stereotypical image of a gentleman.

IS IT WHISKY OR WHISKEY?

Some debate still rages over the historical home of whiskey, whether Ireland or Scotland. Proponents of an Irish origin cite the first documented production license, granted within the Irish district of Bushmills by King James I in 1608. Scottish advocates counter that this information, although historically accurate, is completely irrelevant, as whiskey production logically predated a license to distill whiskey. Indeed, references can be found as early as the 1400s.

History isn't the only subject on which the Irish and Scottish can't see eye to eye. They also disagree when it comes to spelling, with the Irish preferring whiskey to the Scottish whisky. Canadian and Japanese distilleries follow the Scottish convention, while most American whiskey (with the prominent exception of Maker's Mark, Bourbon *Whisky*) aligns with the Irish spelling. Whether you adopt an *"e"* or not in your spelling, make sure to keep an open mind in your drinking.

WHISKEY IS A WORLD AFFAIR

As the alchemy of whiskey-making spread across the world, different regional varieties and methods have emerged based on natural resources and human resourcefulness. Understanding the different types of whiskey available is often one of the biggest stumbling blocks for the new whiskey drinker.

Scotland's Whisky Trail

Oenophiles have long made pilgrimages to the great wine meccas of Napa, Sonoma, and Bordeaux to see where and how their favorite wines are made. Today, whisky lovers can find a similar experience with a trek off the beaten path and onto Scotland's Whisky Trail. The rambling route through the Speyside region of the Highlands is typically covered in about four days and includes visits to some of the most recognized and venerable distilleries in the world. Here are some highlights from the trail:

BENROMACH. Start your tour at the Benromach distillery, the smallest working distillery in Moray. Located on the outskirts of the ancient town of Forres, Benromach is easily recognizable by the distinctive 100-foot-tall red brick chimney rising from the stark white distillery buildings below. Inside, a guided tour, tutored nosing and tasting, and the opportunity to hand-fill your own bottle of single malt await. Benromach is also home to the first fully certified organic single malt.

GLENFIDDICH. One of the few Scotch distilleries still owned and operated by its founding family. Today, Glenfiddich is made using the same ingredients and process originated by founder William Grant in 1839. The Pioneers' Tour offers the chance to taste thirty-year-old whiskies and bottle your own cask-strength Malt Masters Selection, exclusively available through the tour.

THE GLENLIVET. Located in perhaps the most beautiful of distillery settings, the Glenlivet can be found surrounded by rolling green hills dotted with grazing sheep. If you're a Guardian Ambassador, your membership key unlocks the Ambassador Cabinet, granting you access to the special drams in the distillery library.

SPEYSIDE COOPERAGE. Learn all about the traditional art of coopering, the making of oak casks used for storing and aging Scotch whisky. Try your own hand at constructing a cask and then watch the true artisans at work in the only remaining working cooperage in the United Kingdom.

SCOTCH WHISKY. In order to bear the title of Scotch, a whisky must be distilled in a Scottish distillery and matured in oak casks for at least three years. Single-malt Scotch whisky is made from 100 percent malted barley distilled at one distillery. Blended Scotch whisky is a mixture of single malt whisky and grain whisky, usually from a number of different distilleries. Blended-malt Scotch whisky refers to a blend of two or more single-malt whiskies. Any age description on a blended Scotch whisky or blended-malt Scotch whisky must refer to the youngest whisky in the blend.

GRAIN WHISKEY. Grain whiskey is made using at least some grains other than malted barley, including wheat or corn. Most grain whiskey is reserved for blending; however, some especially well-matured batches are bottled and released as single-grain Scotch whisky.

IRISH WHISKEY. Similar to Scotch whisky, but made in Ireland. Irish law mandates that Irish whiskey be distilled in Ireland and matured for at least three years before release. Single malts and blends are both available.

BOURBON. Bourbon must be produced from a mash of at least 51 percent corn but is usually made from 70 to 90 percent corn. The remainder of the mash content is filled with some combination of barley malt, rye, and/or wheat. Law also dictates that bourbon must be matured for at least two years in new, charred, white oak barrels.

TENNESSEE WHISKEY. Tennessee whiskey is bourbon that has been filtered through sugar maple charcoal, a process called the Lincoln County Process.

RYE WHISKEY. Rye whiskey is like bourbon but instead of requiring a mash of at least 51 percent corn, rye whiskey requires a mash of at least 51 percent rye.

CORN WHISKEY. Corn whiskey is made from a fermented mash of at least 80 percent corn. There is no requirement for charred oak barrels and no minimum aging period.

CANADIAN WHISKY. Canadian whisky is a blanket term for any whisky made in Canada. Most Canadian whiskies are a mix of grain whiskey and rye whiskey. To differentiate even further, Canadian law allows up to 9 percent of the final blend to be other flavorings such as sherry, fruit, or foreign whiskey (bourbon is a common additive, for example). Pre-used casks are allowed but the maturation period must be at least three years.

JAPANESE WHISKY. The Japanese follow the Scottish model for whisky production and produce single malts and blended malts to the same specifications.

TOO HARSH . . . TOO DULL . . . JUST RIGHT!

I won't presume to tell you how to drink your whiskey. After all, the only "correct" way to enjoy a wee dram is the way *you* enjoy it most. However, I will tell you how I choose to drink whiskey, as taught to me by a professional Scotch whisky maker.

I will typically order a good whiskey neat (straight) with a side of filtered water. The experience begins with the eyes and nose. I'll swirl the whiskey in the glass and take in the aroma with a few good sniffs. Primed with anticipation, I'll take the first couple sips, neat. I don't swallow good whiskey so much as let it sort of trickle to the back of my throat, spilling over every part of my tongue along its journey. It's at this point when I usually remember why whiskey is referred to as "the breath of angels."

Neat whiskey is often a bit too strong and the harsh "burn" can mask its more complex flavors. Whiskey experts recommend adding a splash of filtered water to open up the aromatics and intricate flavors hidden in the glass. There is actual chemistry behind this reaction, but that's for another time, as right now we're drinking whiskey. It's said that ideally the best water to use is from the same source as the original distillery (some Scottish bars will actually put out little dishes of local spring water) but that's hardly practical; any filtered water should be fine. Don't go overboard; adding just a few drops will usually do. Add some water, swirl, smell, and sip. Add more water to taste, if necessary, and repeat the three S's until your dram is done.

Although it rolls off the tongue easily, ordering whiskey "on the rocks" is not recommended, as the coldness of the ice will dull the flavors and the melted ice will dilute the whiskey. If you prefer your whiskey cold, consider investing in an ice ball press or a set of whiskey stones. The ice ball press creates spherical ice balls rather than ice cubes. A sphere has a much smaller surface area than the equivalent volume of cubed ice, therefore reducing its melt rate. Whiskey stones, on the other hand, are made from nonporous soapstone cubes that can be frozen and used in place of ice with no fear of dilution.

TASTING NOTES

A professional taster will evaluate whiskey using four criteria: appearance, aroma (nose), palate (taste), and finish. You may be anxious to get to the more direct smell and taste of whiskey, but stop for just a second and appreciate its appearance. Note the color, which can provide clues as to the type of cask used (darker amber or copper hues for a sherry cask; golden yellow, honey, or straw hues for a bourbon cask) and length of maturation (generally the older it is the darker it will be). Also take a look at the viscosity of your whiskey. Swirl the whiskey in your glass and observe the "legs" as they drip down the side of the glass. Thick, slow-moving legs usually

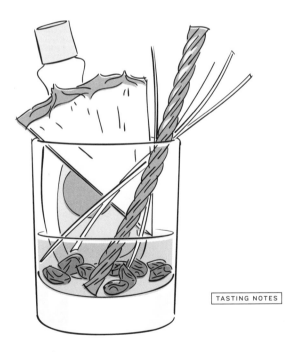

TASTING NOTES

indicate an older whiskey while thin, quick legs are found in younger vintages.

While our tongue can only detect five distinct tastes, our noses can differentiate hundreds of smells. There are eight broad categories of smells commonly found in whiskey (cereal, fruity, floral, peaty, feinty, sulfury, winey, and woody) but don't worry too much about insider jargon. As you sniff, try to associate a word with each smell you detect. If you want a list of common terms to help pinpoint what you smell, take a look at the Whisky Wheel developed by *Whisky Magazine.*

When tasting your whiskey, try to put a specific word or reference to each taste you experience. For example, if you taste an Islay Scotch, you might attribute its characteristic salty flavor to seaweed, ocean air, or sea salt. Again, consult the Whisky Wheel for descriptive adjectives and references if you can't quite nail down what you taste.

Finish refers to how long the whiskey's flavors linger in your mouth. A long finish is generally preferable and the flavors during the finish can often change and evolve so stay tuned, even after you've swallowed.

RECOMMENDATIONS

With so much variation, choosing a whiskey is a highly subjective and difficult, although enjoyable, process. With that preface, here are a few that I enjoy and encourage you to try as well. My criteria for this list were accessibility (in terms of a good introduction for a beginner palate, availability for purchase, and budget) and my own personal taste. *Sláinte!*

BALVENIE DOUBLEWOOD 12-YEAR-OLD

My default recommendation for anyone looking for an introduction to the world of single malts. The Doublewood begins its life in a bourbon cask before graduating to a sherry cask. The result is complex, rich, and sweet with nut and spice notes. The first Scotch I was really able to diagnose and appreciate.

BRUICHLADDICH 10-YEAR-OLD: THE LADDIE TEN

In 2001, a group of intrepid and ambitious investors took over the charismatic but much-neglected Islay distillery. The Laddie Ten is the first wholly controlled release since the Bruichladdich gates were unlocked on that chilly spring morning and the result was well worth the wait. Fresh and bright, with the distinctive maritime tang for which Bruichladdich is known and a finish that lingers longer than some malts twice its age.

YAMAZAKI 12-YEAR-OLD

Bright and crisp, the Yamazaki 12 is a classic Japanese interpretation of whiskey. Starts sweet with a hint of smoke, followed by fruit and finally spice.

GEORGE DICKEL NO. 12

The *other* Tennessee whiskey, and one of the most underrated American whiskeys. Dickel No. 12 is sweeter, lighter, and more complex than its better-known neighbor.

MAKER'S MARK STRAIGHT BOURBON WHISKY

An easy introduction into bourbon as it substitutes wheat for the typically used corn, resulting in a mellower, more delicate character. If you're new to bourbon, try Maker's before jumping to other great brands like Woodford Reserve and Buffalo Trace.

QUESTION TO CONTEMPLATE Do you know the difference between Scotch, bourbon, and Tennessee whiskey? More to the point, does your nose or tongue?

 GENTLEMANLY QUOTE TO REMEMBER "Always carry a flagon of whiskey in case of snakebite and furthermore always carry a small snake."

— W. C. FIELDS

 ACTION STEP Specialty whiskey bars are opening all over, as more and more drinkers discover the joy of whiskey. Find a bar with a good whiskey selection where you can test and experiment without breaking the bank on full bottles. Once you've honed your taste preference over a series of visits, buy a bottle of your new favorite to enjoy at home.

The Gentlemanly Escape

WHILE NOTHING beats a handwritten note or letter for keeping in touch, nothing can match a great trip for creating memories that are worth keeping in touch about. The reality of our normal, day-to-day lives is that they fill up quickly with work obligations, family life, chores, and other commitments. When we do connect with friends, it's often just for minutes at a time. Unless we're really intentional about digging deeper, it's often difficult (and potentially awkward) to move beyond simple small talk to the real substance: our struggles, insecurities, passions, dreams, and aspirations.

As men, we can have difficulty opening up emotionally, but ironically we all crave the life accountability and encouragement that a touch of vulnerability can provide.

I've often found that taking a couple days away with friends is enough to jar us out of our shells and let us get real with one another. For me, the deeper, more meaningful relationships that inevitably emerge from these short trips have made all the difference in negotiating life's ups and downs.

My college friends are an incredibly tight-knit group. In our glory days we pulled off legendary pranks, dominated the intramural sports scene, and established on-campus traditions that still survive today. However, for all our collegiate camaraderie, our postgrad careers have since scattered us to the four winds. Spread across the country from L.A. to New York, Chicago to South Florida, these days it's rare for more than two of us to meet up at any point during a year. That is, until Labor Day rolls around. More than the end of summer, for the twelve of us, Labor Day signals the kickoff of football season and with it our annual fantasy football draft. Each year we gather to stock our virtual rosters, catch up on life, and otherwise fraternize. Tradition dictates that the previous season's winner chooses the following year's draft location, which ensures a fresh experience every time. There's even a trophy on which each champion's name is engraved à la the Stanley Cup. Draft Weekend consistently ranks among the highlights of my year and deepens the strongest of relationships no matter how little we chat on the phone over the previous eleven months.

Here are some tips for planning a great gentlemanly escape of your own:

ADVANCE BOOKING REQUIRED. Ensure solid attendance by locking in plans as far in advance as possible. Get the trip on the books early and you can avoid last-minute excuses

AFFORDABLE ADVENTURES

Here are some ways to save some cash without sacrificing the experience:

RENT A HOUSE. Depending on your group size, renting a house instead of staying at a hotel can be a great way to save money. With a full kitchen you can even cook at home and cut budget-buster eating out. Your bonding experience will also benefit from the extra common space not found in hotel rooms.

CONSIDER A LOCATION WHERE SOMEONE IN YOUR PARTY HAS CONNECTIONS. A corporate box at the stadium or a comped dinner at the latest downtown hot spot might not be that exciting for the host but the groups' collective wallet will thank him nonetheless.

POOL YOUR LOYALTY REWARD PERKS. The road warrior consultant can spring for frequent flyer tickets while the guy with a hoard of hotel points can contribute the accommodations. Those with nothing to offer can pick up the bar tabs, food bills, and activity costs.

AVOID PEAK TRAVEL SEASON. Most places have a peak season and then a couple shoulder months on either side of that peak season that offer as good an experience at much lower prices.

about wives, girlfriends, kids, conflicting plans, or budget constraints. The extra time will also allow you to properly research the location to ensure you're not stuck at a Motel 6 with nothing to do but hit up the local Starbucks.

GET OFF THE GRID. The next few days are all about the fellow gentlemen with whom you're escaping. Leave the work smartphone and laptop at home. Set expectations with family and friends that you'll be incommunicado except for emergencies. Don't check email, get off Facebook; leave the digital world and be fully present in the physical moment.

ACTIVITIES, PLEASE. Shared experiences create stories that cement themselves into memories that last for years and truly deepen friendships. While you'll want to leave some downtime just to relax and hang out, make sure that your trip also includes plenty of planned activities that take advantage of your location and the fact that you have a large group together.

COMPETITION BREEDS CAMARADERIE. For some reason, probably evolutionary, many men are predisposed to competition. Some good-natured, low-stakes competition can go a long way toward heightening a gentlemen's escape. Consider upping the ante on your male bonding by adding an element of competition to your activities. My friends and I often create a list of events at the start of Draft Weekend, dubbed the Hubris Challenge, ranging from board games and sporting activities to social challenges. Keeping score throughout the weekend keeps everyone engaged and having fun.

Trip planning can be as easy as simply choosing a destination, but if you want to tailor your trip to a specific theme or interest, here are some getaway ideas for inspiration:

THE OUTDOOR SPORTSMAN. If you think heaven will smell like spent shotgun shells and sound like a line gently cast over a bubbling brook, head for the unspoiled beauty of the Smoky Mountains or another world-class fly fishing, sport shooting destination. Trade in "up to your elbows in paperwork" for "knee-deep in trout-filled streams" and take out your pent-up frustration with office politics on some unsuspecting skeet. Then retire for a night of arguments over who landed the biggest river monster or shattered the most clay with the aged whiskey, overstuffed leather chairs, and crackling fireplace of a luxury sportsman lodge.

THE RETIRED ATHLETE. Follow your favorite sports team to training camp or spring training. Get an up-close look at your team as it gears up for the season and offer encouragement at a time when your passion as a fan can be singularly appreciated by the team. Since many teams choose to train in smaller cities and towns, you can emulate your favorite players in pickup games by day then buy them a round at the local restaurants and watering holes by night.

THE DRIVING ENTHUSIAST. Spend a few days bonding at 150 mph while enrolled at a high-performance driving school. Most racetracks offer schools for all skill levels. Rent a couple good sports cars and hit a beautiful roadway.

THE ADVENTURE SURVIVALIST. Literally get off the grid and head out into the great wide open. With nothing but your friends, the gear on your back, and the beautiful solitude of nature for company, you'll be surprised how quickly you can get to the core of who you are and what matters most. Plus, you'll experience one of the great mysteries of life: how a long day's trek in the backcountry can turn freeze-dried food into Michelin star-worthy gourmet fare.

QUESTION TO CONTEMPLATE When was the last time you got away with just the guys, no girlfriends, wives, or kids? Not a day trip to the ballpark or a quick nine holes at the club, but a full-on, overnight MAN WEEKEND. Think about how taking a trip together can forge and strengthen the bonds of brotherhood in your male friendships.

 GENTLEMANLY QUOTE TO REMEMBER "Never go on trips with anyone you do not love."

— Ernest Hemingway

 ACTION STEP Take the initiative on organizing a guys' trip for your friends. Take charge in coordinating a time, location, and activities, because if you don't do it, no one will. Use the recommendations and advice in this chapter for inspiration.

Date Night Might

ON APRIL 11, 1917, while World War I was raging through Europe, young love was raging through the U.S. Legation office in Bern, Switzerland. A junior diplomat and eventual head of the CIA, twenty-four-year-old Allen Dulles, had finally landed a date with longtime crush Helene Herzog following an almost nine-year courtship. As Dulles was closing his office early in anticipation of his romantic rendezvous, he received a rather inopportune phone call. On the other line was a Russian revolutionary who insisted on meeting to deliver some extremely important, time-sensitive information. Dulles, however, refused to cancel his date, instead informing the caller that any meeting had to wait until the morning.

The man protested that the next day would be too late, but the lovesick Dulles was unmoved. After all, Dulles had waited nine years for his date with Ms. Herzog; surely the information in question could wait a few hours, right?

History doesn't tell us how the date went but we do know that while the date was happening, Vladimir Lenin boarded the famous sealed train that took him and his conspirators from Switzerland to St. Petersburg and on to lead the Bolshe-

---

FIRST DATE DO'S

Clean up. Dress to impress. Pay. There are a lot of no-brainer do's on a first date, but here are a few less common tips for your first romantic rendezvous:

• Don't be early for the pickup. Normally I live by the "five minutes early is on time" philosophy, but when it comes to a date, most women like to use every last minute to get ready. Don't surprise her early when she's still in sweats and half-finished makeup.

• Set dress expectations in advance. If you're going hiking, spare your date the embarrassment of showing up in a little black dress and heels by providing a heads-up a few days in advance.

• Break the physical barrier early. Pair a hug with a "You look fantastic!" at the beginning of the date and she'll feel more comfortable showing her own affection, making your job of reading signals for how the date is going much easier.

• Complimentary is complementary. Compliment your date, of course, but also speak kindly of others and you'll project a sense of positivity that is positively charming.

---

vik Russian Revolution. Lenin had intended to pass along a secret message to President Woodrow Wilson to give advance notice of his plans, and to discuss the events that would follow. The conversation between president and revolutionary never materialized, and under Lenin's influence, Russia went on to withdraw from WWI, endure a bloody civil war, and re-emerge as the communist USSR. We'll never know, but if not for Dulles's date, perhaps the entire course of the twentieth century might have played out differently.

Here's how to prepare if you ever land a date worthy of sacrificing your job, national security, and global stability.

SAVE THE DATE

Before you go on a date, you need to get a date.

When it comes to asking someone on a date, there's no secret sauce; initiate conversation, and once you've built a bit of a connection, just ask politely and directly. If the answer is no then let it go, at least for the moment. No matter what you've seen in the movies, chances are unlikely that you're charming enough to convince an on-the-spot change of heart with a witty quip or charismatic plea.

"MEET ME AT CENTER ICE"

Save grand gestures until after you've built some rapport, and you know the statement will be well-received. In college I once had a buddy sneak me into the PA booth at a hockey game. Partly out of romantic idealism and partly on a dare, I asked the prettiest girl in school to meet me at center ice after the game if she was interested in going out on a date. After the game I was left standing alone like an idiot. I later came to find out that it wasn't me, but the public announcement and embarrassment that had turned her off. She would have said yes had I simply asked her out, face to face.

DATE PLANNER

A gentleman is never shy about showing initiative and taking the lead. Especially in the early days of a relationship, it's your responsibility to tackle the planning so that your companion is free to simply relax and enjoy the date. The first couple of dates should be all about getting to know one another, so focus on activities that facilitate and heighten conversation. Including an activity of some kind can help remove pressure, but don't opt for something completely non-social (not to mention uncreative) like a movie.

As relationships progress, dates start to become more about developing and deepening connections. At this point, you should have a good idea of the interests and passions of your date, and your plans should reflect them. Remember that sharing a new experience or overcoming a fear with someone instantly forms strong relational bonds. You can use this relational psychology to your advantage by exploring new foods, cutting a rug in an Intro to Zouk dance class, or staring down acrophobia by jumping out of a plane together.

DATE NIGHT ETIQUETTE

While walking, try to position yourself on the street side of the sidewalk (a throwback to a time when water, mud, and other unsavory mess was routinely splashed by passing carriages). If you cross a street and suddenly find yourself on the "wrong" side, don't worry about exchanging places unless you can do so unobtrusively. And should safety concerns dictate that you break the rule, by all means, do so.

CREATIVE DATES FOR ANY MATE

Here are some suggestions for breaking out of the predictable dinner-and-a-movie rut at any stage of a relationship:

• BE TOURISTS FOR A DAY. Embrace the crowds and mingle with the out-of-towners for once. Visit local tourist traps you normally avoid; it's surprising how a different mind-set can completely change your experience!

• BRING THINGS TO A BOIL. A cooking class is a fun and interactive date with a (hopefully) delicious ending. If there isn't a culinary school in your area, check out community colleges or local restaurants.

• VOLUNTEER CHEER. Make a difference in your community and demonstrate your gentlemanly character. The good feelings you'll both get are sure to spill over into your relationship.

• GET HOT AND SWEATY. If you're both fit and active types, attend yoga, spinning, or CrossFit class together. You'll release some feel-good endorphins and work up an appetite for a healthy, post-workout brunch.

• X MARKS THE SPOT. Experience the excitement of finding buried treasure with a geocaching date. All you need is a portable GPS device, online clues, and an adventurous spirit.

• JAZZ IT UP. Ignite your passion in the atmosphere of an intimate, dimly lit jazz club. Between the sultry music and your whispered communication, your hearts will be dancing as much as the notes.

• RIPE FOR THE PICKING. Grab a blanket and go pick whatever fruit is in season: strawberries in late spring, peaches in summer, apples in autumn. Sit and talk on your blanket while enjoying the sweet fruit of your labor.

As a general rule, when approaching a door, discreetly step forward and open the door for your companion. Always open doors unless doing so requires making a scene of some kind. If your date clearly reaches a door ahead of you and starts to open it, grab the edge of the door and subtly take over the task.

Always seat your date facing the room, never into a wall. This placement allows your date to see and be seen by the rest of the room while limiting the visual distractions that might divert your attention from your companion.

When you get to a table, pull your date's chair away from the table, and then gently hold it as your date sits down. At the end of the meal, gently pull the chair back as your date pushes it away while standing up. This is an easy and almost universally well-accepted gesture of chivalry. Proceed without hesitation.

Ordering at a restaurant presents the gentleman on the town with a high-risk, high-reward opportunity. Some dates are honored by and attracted to the take-charge confidence and courtesy you exhibit when ordering for them. However, some prefer to order for themselves and may even interpret your chivalrous intentions as arrogance. If you're sure the person you're with will appreciate the gesture, ask what your date would like and when the waiter comes, confidently place the order for both of you.

Traditionally, men should stand whenever a woman approaches or leaves a table. While this practice has largely fallen by the wayside, most women still appreciate the gesture. This move must be done with confidence; hesitant attempts will inevitably result in awkward moments. However, when executed well, "The Stand" will help you stand out as a true gentleman.

DON'T BE SCARED OF "OVERDOING IT"

My wife and I were recently at an event where we were asked to participate in an icebreaker game modeled after *The New-lywed Game.* In response to the question "What is the most romantic thing your husband has ever done?" there were audible groans and heckling from the men in attendance as my wife recounted our first anniversary together. Somehow my action, not their inaction, made them look bad, and it was my fault that "bringing home flowers once" didn't score huge points on the romance front.

What I've come to realize is that many men deliberately avoid elaborate romantic gestures out of fear of setting the bar, and future expectations, too high. It's not that these men don't want to do something special for their someone special, it's that they don't want special to become expected, and therefore taken for granted. The problem is, in most relationships, this logic is completely flawed.

While I haven't done much to match the private plane ride to the Hamptons for our first anniversary dinner, my wife has never used that night as a counterpoint to bemoan my subsequent lack of romanticism to the same standard. In fact, the opposite is true; she remembers that night often, and fondly, and still tells the story as excitedly as she did the morning afterwards. Gentlemen, I implore you to break the romantic status quo. Go over the top, even if just once, and you'll experience the pure joy of making someone special truly feel that way.

QUESTION TO CONTEMPLATE Is the thought and effort you put into your dating life consistent with your affection for the person you're dating, whether on a second date or a thirtieth anniversary? Don't extraordinary relationships deserve extraordinary celebration?

GENTLEMANLY QUOTE TO REMEMBER "How can a woman be expected to be happy with a man who insists on treating her as if she were a perfectly normal human being?"

— Oscar Wilde

ACTION STEP No matter what relationship stage you're in, plan and execute an exceptional date for an exceptional person.

30

Work Out Like a Navy SEAL

MY BEST FRIEND, and best man at my wedding, is in Navy SEAL training. Hanging out with him is an exercise in humility. This was especially true when he led me and four other city slickers up into the ten-foot-deep snow of Yosemite's high country for a long weekend, bachelor party adventure. The trip was akin to the episode of the adventure show *Man vs. Wild* in which outdoor survivalist Bear Grylls takes comedic actor Will Ferrell into the wilderness, only we were less prepared than Ferrell. Under Jason's guidance we fished our dinner out of frozen lakes, climbed mountain ridges, snowshoed across glistening meadows, and didn't see a soul for four days. It was spectacular, but I'm sure that without Jason, we would have died out there.

Outdoorsmanship isn't the only area in which Jason puts me to shame. His fitness is legendary. In a couple moments of ill-fated, Odysseus-like hubris, I attempted to keep pace with Jason during his notorious high-intensity workouts. Let's just say things did not end well. As the tip of the U.S. Navy's special warfare spear, SEALs pride themselves on elite, functional fitness. In other words, SEALs were dominating CrossFit workouts before it was trendy. I push away from my desk and pull a hamstring.

WHY FITNESS MATTERS FOR THE AVERAGE, NON-SEAL GENTLEMAN

Becoming a better man requires a lot of internally focused work: broadening of knowledge, development of character, and cultivation of good intentions. However, exercise of the body is just as important as exercise of the mind. Living life to its full potential requires good health. It's difficult to go to the symphony, open doors, enjoy Scotch, fix a car, or host a dinner party in poor health. Furthermore, a gentleman greatly benefits from a sharp mind when engaged in the hard work of self-reflection and character building. And we all know that a sound body leads to a sharp mind (not to mention a better-fitting suit).

Modern life is sedentary life. Part of the gentleman manifesto is living with intention, and today exercise requires more intention than ever before. So even if you are more likely to be found behind a desk than behind enemy lines, fitness still matters. If your physical fitness routine needs a jump-start, give the following workouts a shot.

THE TRACK WORKOUT

For SEALs, workout portability is important. Since SEALs

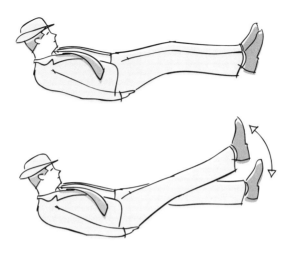

FLUTTER KICK

travel often and may not be in the same place for long, a workout that doesn't require equipment and can be done anywhere is highly valued. For this reason, body weight exercises like push-ups and flutter kicks form the core of SEAL physical training (PT).

The goal of this particular workout is to see your performance improve over time as you work at the individual elements and generally increase your fitness. On your first time out, this workout will probably be pretty tough. You may need to break up the push-up reps or walk occasionally on the run sections — and that's okay. As your fitness increases you'll be able to complete the training as described without breaks, and you'll watch your completion times plummet. Remember to record your training times so you can track your progress. If at any point you want to increase the repetitions, go for it!

Complete sequentially against a continuously running clock, as quickly as possible:

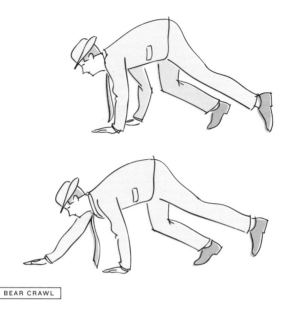

BEAR CRAWL

- Run/jog one mile (four laps on a standard track)
- 50 push-ups
- 50 crunches
- 50-yard prisoner lunges
- 50 four-count flutter kicks
- 50-yard bear crawl
- 50 crunches
- 50 push-ups
- Run/jog one mile

THE SEAL PST

The PST or Physical Screening Test is the benchmark fitness test for Navy SEALs. If you want to see how you stack up against some of the most elite athletes in the world, give it a shot. The target scores indicate competitive marks for actual

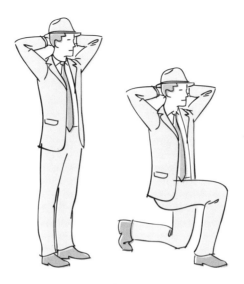

SEALs; if you can hit them, congratulations, you're in great company.

- Swim 500 yards using breast and/or side stroke in less than II minutes and 30 seconds (target less than 9 minutes)

REST I0 MINUTES

- Complete at least 42 push-ups in 2 minutes (target 90+ repetitions)

REST 2 MINUTES

- Complete at least 50 sit-ups in 2 minutes (target 90+ repetitions)

REST 2 MINUTES

- Complete at least 8 pull-ups (target 20+ repetitions)

REST I0 MINUTES

- Run I.5 miles in less than II minutes (target less than 9 minutes)

QUESTION TO CONTEMPLATE What does fitness have to do with modern gentlemanliness? What does your fitness level say about you?

 GENTLEMANLY QUOTE TO REMEMBER "It is exercise alone that supports the spirits, and keeps the mind in vigor."

— Cicero

 ACTION STEP Complete the Track Workout or Navy SEAL PST in place of your normal workout. If possible, enlist a workout partner. You'll motivate each other and allow each of you to focus on the exercises without worrying about checking form, counting reps, or keeping time.

Appendix ~ The Thirty Action Steps

1 TWENTY THINGS EVERY GENTLEMAN SHOULD OWN
Take an inventory against the list and consider buying or upgrading an item.

2 A CLASSICAL (MUSIC) EDUCATION
Explore the list of musical recommendations.

3 A GENTLEMAN THROWS A PARTY
Throw a fantastic bash.

4 A MACRO VIEW ON MICROBREWS
Organize a craft beer tasting.

5 A MORNING ROUTINE FOR DAILY DOMINATION
Commit to a week of early rising and structured mornings.

6 BOOKS EVERY GENTLEMAN SHOULD READ
Read one of the recommended titles with a fellow gentleman.

7 THE CONFIDENT CONVERSATIONALIST
Attempt a conversation in which you don't talk about yourself at all.

8 DATE NIGHT MIGHT

Plan and execute an exceptional date for an exceptional person.

9 DELIVER A TOAST WORTH DRINKING TO

Find an excuse to offer a toast with your next drink.

10 DINE LIKE ROYALTY: ETIQUETTE AT THE DINNER TABLE

Evaluate your eating habits by eating in front of a mirror or video camera.

11 FIND A MENTOR, BE A MENTOR

Think about what you want from a mentor and seek one out.

12 FROM DANDY TO HANDY: EMERGENCY CAR RESCUE

Practice changing a tire in your driveway.

13 HOW TO BUILD AND MAINTAIN A POWERFUL NETWORK

Plan something to deepen a meaningful relationship.

14 iGENT: ETIQUETTE FOR THE DIGITAL AGE

Audit your online presence.

15 MANDATE TO CREATE

Create something!

16 **THE MAN-ICURE**

Evaluate your hygiene and make changes accordingly.

17 **MIX A SPECIALTY COCKTAIL...AND MAKE SOME MEMORIES**

Mix a signature drink for your next dinner party, poker game, or date night.

18 **PERSONAL PHILOSOPHY FOR PRACTICAL PURPOSE**

Evaluate *what* you believe and *why*.

19 **POETRY FOR MEN**

Find a poem that resonates with you and carry it with you until it has been committed to memory.

20 **READY, SET, GO-ALS! THE GENTLEMAN'S BUCKET LIST**

Write your own personal bucket list.

21 **START AN HONORABLE GENTLEMAN'S CLUB**

Join or start a club.

22 **THE COURAGE TO ENCOURAGE**

Call someone who could benefit from some encouragement.

23 **THE GENTLEMANLY ESCAPE**

Organize a guy's trip for your friends.

24 **THE PROPER CARE AND FEEDING OF DRESS SHOES**
Shine your own shoes.

25 **THE PROPER TECHNIQUE FOR IRONING A DRESS SHIRT**
Iron a shirt for yourself or someone else.

26 **THE SARTORIAL MATCHMAKER: COMBINATIONS THAT WORK, FOR WORK**
Combine two or more elements from your closet that you've never worn together before.

27 **WELL PACKED: INSIDE A GENTLEMAN'S TRAVEL BAG**
Practice the folding techniques and use them on your next trip.

28 **WHISK(E)Y: THE WATER OF LIFE**
Find a specialty whiskey bar and order something you've never had before.

29 **WHY THE TIE SHOULD NEVER DIE**
Wear a tie somewhere unexpected.

30 **WORK OUT LIKE A NAVY SEAL**
Complete the Track Workout or Navy SEAL PST during your next workout.

Acknowledgements

Many thanks to Steve Mockus, who championed this project with great enthusiasm and honed my vision with his insightful editing.

Thank you to my wife, Jenny, for her unwavering support and encouragement throughout the writing of this book. Thank you to my father for the constant childhood reminders to "act like an officer and a gentleman" that have become ingrained in my character, and to my mother for lovingly holding me to the highest standards.

Thank you to Saras Sarasvathy, who empowered me to turn my entrepreneurial dreams into reality. And huge thanks to Brett Nicol; whose indomitable spirit, energy, and optimism launched Forgetful Gentleman and made this book possible.

And, of course, a big thank you to the thousands of forgetful gentlemen around the world, many of whom contributed comments, suggestions, and ideas that influenced this book and my life.

Cheers!

About the Author

NATHAN TAN is founder and CEO of Forgetful Gentleman, helping the modern man become the best possible version of himself. As the original Forgetful Gentleman, he knows all about the challenges of turning good intentions into action and has been profiled by Bloomberg/Businessweek, NBC, and British Airways Business Life. He has an MBA from the Darden School at the University of Virginia and lives with his family in New York City.

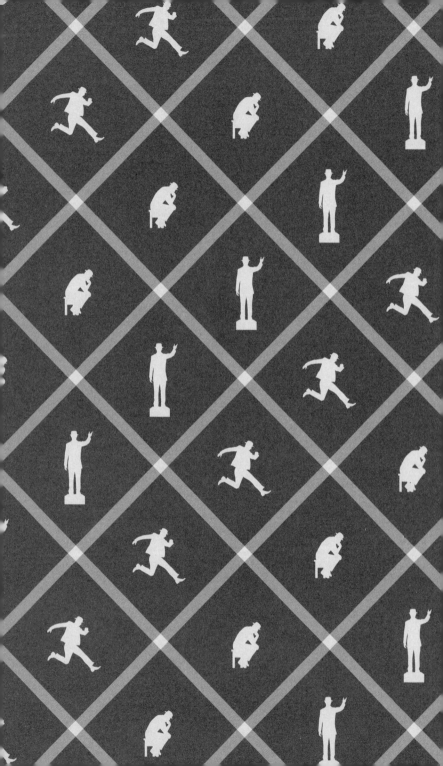